Perspectives in Gynaecology and Obstetrics

Perspectives in Gynaecology and Obstetrics

Selected Plenary Papers presented at the
XIV European Congress of Gynaecologists and Obstetricians,
Granada, Spain, September 1999

EBCOG

EAGO

Edited by
Francisco González Gomez
and
Santiago Palacios

The Parthenon Publishing Group
International Publishers in Medicine, Science & Technology

NEW YORK LONDON

Library of Congress
Cataloging-in-Publication Data
Data available on request

British Library
Cataloguing in Publication Data
Data available on request

ISBN 1-85070-774-X

Published in the USA by
The Parthenon Publishing Group Inc.
One Blue Hill Plaza
PO Box 1564, Pearl River
New York 10965, USA

Published in the UK and Europe by
The Parthenon Publishing Group Limited
Casterton Hall, Carnforth
Lancs. LA6 2LA, UK

Typeset by AMA DataSet Ltd., Preston, UK
Printed and bound in Spain by
T.G. Hostench, S.A.

Contents

Gynaecological malignancies

Pelvic pain

Postgraduate training

List of principal contributors

S. Alexander
Université Libre de Bruxelles
École de Salut Public
Route de Lennik, 808
B-1070 Bruxelles
Belgium

M. Barata
Rua du Campo Grande
Lisboa
Portugal

P. Barri
Institut Dexeus
Paseo Bonanova, 67
Barcelona 08017
Spain

M. W. Beckmann
Department of Obstetrics and Gynecology
Heinrich-Heine Universität
Moorenstrasse 5
40225 Düsseldorf
Germany

M. Brincat
Faculty of Medicine & Surgery
Medical School
University of Malta
Gwardamangia
Malta

S. Greggi
Department of Obstetrics and Gynecology
Catholic University of Sacred Heart
Largo Agostino Gemelli 8
00168 Rome
Italy

F. Goffinet
CH Int. Leon Touhidjian
Université Paris
123, bd de Port-Royal
75679 Paris Cedex 14
France

F. González Gomez
University of Granada
Granda
Spain

J. Lansac
University Hospital Bretonneau
Tours Cedex
F-37004
France

L. Nappi
Institute of Obstetrics and Gynecology
University of Bari
Villa Simonelli
San Paolo Belsito (NA)
80030
Italy

M. Neves-e-Castro
Av. António Augusto de Aguiar
24, 2°Dto–1050-016 Lisbon
Portugal

F. Nunes
Rua Nuno Almada
Botehlo, 16–3°B
Almada 2800
Portugal

S. Palacios
Instituto Professor Palacios
Madrid
Spain

E. Petri
Department of Obstetrics and Gynecology
University of Rostock
Wismarsche Str. 397
D-19049 Schwerin
Germany

F. J. Regateiro
Service of Genetics
University of Coimbra
3049 Coimbra codex
Portugal

P. Reginald
Princess Christian Hospital
12 Clarence Road
Windsor
Berkshire SL4 5AG
UK

J. G. Schenker
Department of Obstetrics and Gynecology
Hadassah University Hospital
P.O. Box 12000
Jerusalem 91120
Israel

D. W. Sturdee
Department of Obstetrics and Gynaecology
Solihul Hospital
Lode Lane
Solihul
West Midlands
UK

J. M. van Geelen
St. Anna Hospital
Postbus 10
5340 BE Oss
The Netherlands

Preface

This book is a selection of some of the key plenary papers contributed by eminent European health professionals to the 14th Congress of the European Association of Gynaecologists and Obstetricians (EAGO) and the European Board and College of Obstetricians and Gynaecologists (EBCOGs) held in Granada (Spain) as we approach the 21st century (September–October 1999). Some other key papers presented at the Congress may be published in appropriate journals at a later date.

The major aims of EAGO are to promote active scientific thinking, as well as to consider the ethical and social implications of current gynaecological and obstetric practice. This spirit emerges from the pages of this book, in which the research and clinical experience of the authors are offered in order to provide a useful tool to improve the knowledge of our discipline. The highly interesting topics covered here will be an updated source of information, especially for our younger colleagues. Furthermore, we hope the work that is presented in this book will stimulate the reader to maintain a high degree of active commitment aimed at achieving high standards in the practice of gynaecology and obstetrics in all European countries.

We would like to mention that EAGO is very pleased to have the contribution of eminent members of EBCOGs for the first time. The efforts of this young association to improve quality training in obstetrics and gynaecology deserve our greatest respect and support, as well as emphatic applause. Everyone in our discipline will be delighted to know the steps that EBCOGs and the European Network of Trainees in Obstetrics and Gynaecology are making in order to ensure comparable and high-quality training in European countries.

To achieve and maintain a high quality of life throughout an individual's lifespan is a collective ideal world-wide, and represents our hopes at the end of this century. Health professionals are now involved more than ever in the task of helping their patients to obtain this ideal. Most of the topics covered here, from reproductive life to the postmenopausal period, deal with the prevention of disease and the best means of maintaining quality of life.

Topics of current great interest, such as strategies to fight against sterility and infertility, are followed by discussions on the long-term risks for mother and child associated with infertility treatments. Moreover, results are presented from studies on the possible genetic risks associated with *in vitro* fertilization/intracytoplasmic sperm injection (IVF/ICSI), as well as on the possible association between assisted reproductive techniques and gynaecological malignancies.

The role of prematurity markers is also discussed, as well as the role of available tests to determine fetal well-being.

With regard to the health of postmenopausal women (an increasing proportion of the population), the effects of estrogenic deficiency on the cardiovascular system, bones and central nervous system are reviewed. The available evidence on the role that hormone replacement therapy might have on the risk of developing cardiovascular diseases, osteoporosis and central nervous system diseases is presented in order to discuss the benefits that might be obtained by the use of this therapy. Nevertheless, many women are still reluctant to use this treatment and thus compliance is low. Continuous combined hormone replacement therapy seems to be a therapeutic scheme that could improve compliance, and thus a review of the available studies on this regime can be found in this book.

Current topics in oncology are also covered, especially with regard to the advances made in this field. The role that selective estrogen receptor modulators might have on the prevention of breast cancer is an interesting subject that deserves great attention; ongoing clinical trials will allow an assessment to be made of the benefits offered by these compounds.

On the other hand, the clinical implications of molecular screening in gynaecological cancers are discussed and special attention is paid to the practical problems that might arise during the identification and management of high-risk patients. In addition, an interesting chapter on Fallopian tube tumors is included.

Urinary incontinence is another topic covered here because it has a high prevalence in postmenopausal women and might affect their quality of life. It appears that it is possible to identify women at risk of developing urinary incontinence. There is an interesting discussion on the role that Cesarean section might have as a preventive measure against urinary incontinence in pregnant women at high risk of developing this disorder in the future. Furthermore, there are other discussions concerning surgical techniques for the treatment of urogynaecological disorders.

We would like to point out that a scientific congress is organized not only to exchange information and to reinforce the sense of belonging to a group, but also, in our modest opinion, to stimulate scientific curiosity and encourage individual effort every day to improve the knowledge of our discipline to which we are dedicating a great part of our lives. We hope that this book will encourage you to keep your mind open to the scientific advances that will appear in future years.

Finally, we would like, on behalf of EAGO and EBCOGs, to express our most sincere gratitude to the authors for their invaluable contributions to the Congress and to this book.

Francisco González Gomez, MD, PhD
President of the Organizing Committee

Santiago Palacios, MD, PhD
General Secretary of the Organizing Committee

Obstetrics

1

Premature markers: a reality?

F. Goffinet

CLASSICAL MARKERS AVAILABLE

For the past 30 years many markers have been used to identify patients at high risk for preterm delivery. The main criteria are socioeconomic factors, past history and symptoms observed during pregnancy (e.g. hemorrhage, uterine contractions and cervical modifications). Scores have been designed to use these criteria in clinical practice. Some countries developed prenatal care for the prevention of prematurity for the whole population and not only for those women who were well informed and using medical care (women at lower risk than others). The incidence of prematurity is lower in these countries than in those without developed prenatal care; however, prematurity, particularly extreme prematurity, has increased over the past few years in all countries. Many factors can explain this increase, but we will not discuss all of them. One example is that the identification of high-risk women is not as good in clinical practice as reported in studies. A second point is that interventions after screening do not seem to be effective.

OBJECTIVES OF NEW MARKERS

Recently, many new markers have been evaluated to improve screening (transvaginal ultrasound cervical measurement, fibronectin, bacterial vaginosis, salivary estriol, etc.). It is not certain that the high predictive value reported in these studies would be the same in clinical practice. To recommend the systematic use of these new markers in addition to existing markers, several conditions are required. Because of its systematic use, the new test must be simple to perform, have good reproducibility and not be too expensive. Moreover, its predictive value must be higher than that of current markers and effective management must be available after screening.

TREATMENT AFTER SCREENING?

Two treatments could be offered to women at high risk for preterm delivery. The first is a symptomatic management when preterm labor occurs. Almost all cases of spontaneous preterm delivery are preceded by preterm labor. Therefore, whatever the cause of preterm labor, we will always need a symptomatic intervention which can be beneficial. Controlled randomized trials on home uterine activity monitoring and education showed an increase in the early diagnosis of preterm labor and a reduction in preterm delivery in a high-risk population. Even this symptomatic management (education of women and contact with midwives, bedrest, tocolysis) does not decrease the incidence of prematurity, but it can decrease the neonatal consequences of extreme prematurity. Indeed, tocolysis results in a mean prolongation of gestation of 2 days, with the possibility of giving corticoids and organizing an *in utero* transfer to a level III center.

The second treatment is etiological and could be very effective in preventive and in curative treatment. This management could be focused on populations representing a small proportion of all preterm deliveries, and could include cerclage of the cervix in cases of cervical incompetence and treatment with antibiotics if subclinical infection was diagnosed. Therefore, a particular method of etiological management will never be effective for the entire population. However, for these specific etiological groups, it is probably the most effective procedure.

CONCLUSION

The objective of the new markers is two-fold. We need etiological markers and symptomatic markers to propose effective management for the entire population. Current markers are not etiological and their predictive value for preterm delivery is lower in practice than in experimental studies. Maybe improvement in clinical practice is possible with better organization of prenatal care.

New markers cannot be used in practice before the evaluation of their impact on prematurity, otherwise physicians will multiply the use of markers, in combination or not, without benefit for women. Improvement must be directed, first, at an application more effective than existing screening and prenatal care, second, at finding interventions following screening that are more efficacious than the existing ones, and, finally, to the use of new markers, both etiological and symptomatic.

2

Fetal movements and fetus behavior as tests of fetal well-being

S. Alexander, M. Delcroix, F. Puech and the Multicenter Fetal Movement Testing – France Group

'And the children struggled together within her; and she (Rebecca) said, "If it be so, why am I thus?" '

Genesis: 25, 22

'Premature labour should be induced on the mother feeling that the movements of the children are less strong'

Playfair, 1884

INTRODUCTION

Fetal movements and fetal behavior are two sides of the same coin: motor activity of the unborn child. The former has been of interest for centuries, whilst the latter has only been accessible since the advent of ultrasound. Both have been regarded as markers of fetal health, though formal evaluation is often lacking.

The two tests which have been best evaluated are, first, the subjective counting of fetal movements by the mother, and, second, the fetal biophysical profile, which is achieved using a combination of ultrasound and fetal heart-rate monitoring. Two more aspects of fetal activity need to be mentioned: movements elicited by acoustic stimulation and global motor activity behavior studies.

The present chapter will be divided into two sections: the first on maternal perception of fetal movements and the second on other techniques (biophysical profile, acoustic stimulation and fetal behavior). All sections will comprise a review of the literature. The section on fetal movements will also include unpublished data from the MFMT-F (Multicenter Fetal Movement Testing–France) study.

Fetal movement counts (maternal perception of fetal movements)

Maternal perception of fetal movements is reported by Rebecca in Genesis: when pregnant with twins, she enquires about 'the struggling in her womb'.

In the English language, there is a verb 'to quicken', the definition of which is: '(of a woman) to reach a stage in pregnancy when movements of the foetus can be felt'[1]; in French there is no such verb and it is necessary to use a roundabout expression ['sentir les mouvements du bébé' (to feel the movements of the baby)] to express the same situation. Reference to the Bible and the existence of a verb in its own right seem to provide sufficient evidence that the perception of fetal movements is one of the oldest known signs of a live pregnancy.

The recommendation that this perception be used as an obstetrical risk marker can be traced to at least a century ago. Playfair[2] advised induction of labor in the presence of decreasing fetal movements. During the 20th century, the standard routine for antenatal care includes systematic enquiry about quickening, although seldom in terms of quantity of the movements. In 1973, two obstetrical teams separately published observations suggesting that formal counting of fetal movements by the mother could be an efficient test of fetal well-being[3,4]. There are at least four self-evident theoretical benefits of this method:

(1) It is cheap, requiring only a pencil, paper and a watch.

(2) It can be repeated daily, allowing close surveillance.

(3) It is entrusted to the mother, encouraging responsible self-surveillance and partnership between caregiver and patient.

(4) It enhances early bonding between mother and child[5].

Methods of formal counting belong to either the fixed-count or the fixed-time approach. In the fixed-count format, women count until they have felt a fixed number of kicks and the threshold is a duration of time above which there is cause for alarm. Probably the most popular fixed-count format is the 'count to ten', in which women count until they have felt ten kicks and there is alarm if ten kicks are not felt in 10 h. In the fixed-time format, women count for a fixed number of minutes and the threshold is the number of kicks which is considered to be the minimal acceptable for that duration of time. A surprising observation is that a great diversity of schedules have been published, both for counting regimens and for thresholds. Reviews of these various schedules can be found[6,7]. These variations did not, in their time, seem to impair the dissemination of the test.

Fetal movement counting was initially described for high-risk pregnancies and designed as an additional tool for detecting deterioration in an already compromised pregnancy. It was later suggested that extending counting to all pregnancies might help to tackle the problem of unexpected fetal deaths in apparently normal pregnancies.

Materials and methods

A general review of the literature was performed pertaining to the count of fetal movements in relation to three topics:

(1) Counting as a test of well-being;

(2) Feasibility and compliance;

(3) Ideal counting regimen and extrapolation of counts to daily activity.

This review aims to be complete in relation to these three topics. Feasibility and compliance were also assessed from our own unpublished data in two studies on fetal movement counts:

(1) The Multicenter Fetal Movement Trial (MFMT) performed in Belgium, Ireland, Sweden, the UK and the USA was designed to evaluate the effectiveness of maternal counting. Details of the methodology and global results have been published[8]. We used the data of the Belgian participation to give a description of feasibility and compliance aspects.

(2) The Multicenter Fetal Movement Testing–France (MFMT-F), performed in seven units in France, was an *ad hoc* study designed to assess the feasibility of fetal

movement counting regimens. This study was partly generated by the questions raised by the MFMT study described above. It was an observational study, simply aimed at assessing feasibility and an optimal schedule.

Piloting

In France, formal fetal movement counting is not largely used; when it is used, it is restricted to high-risk pregnancies. The implementation of formal counting introduces a totally new scheme to the antenatal clinics, both in terms of workload and attitudes. This situation prompted a 3-month pilot phase, during which counting was introduced into the antenatal clinics of the collaborating units.

Study phase: instruction to women and rate of participation

Seven hospitals participated in the study phase. All women attending the antenatal clinics were asked to register fetal movements, starting as early as the 28th week. A fixed-time approach was selected. In the first months of the study, women were asked to count for 1 h three times a day. In the second part of the study, women were asked to count for 30 min, also three times a day. During both periods, women were asked to fill in their chart each time they counted and also to write out in full all medications they were taking. No instructions were given regarding thresholds for normal or abnormal counts, as the aim of the study was to establish normal values. Counts were anonymous and women were encouraged to write down any personal comments prompted by the counting procedure. Only women who delivered charts for at least two complete weeks were included for analysis. This left a total of 26 469 counts in 443 pregnancies. Of these, 343 had counted for 1 h three times a day and 100 had counted for 30 min three times a day.

Statistical analysis

Statistical analysis was performed on SPSS/PC+. Comparisons of results in the different counting situations were made using the Wilcoxon–Mann–Whitney non-parametric test, because of the non-Gaussian distribution of the counts. Comparisons were made between medians and lower centiles for the different durations of counts. Because many of the early studies used average numbers of counts, these were also computed, exclusively for comparison purposes.

Computation of a 'continuation rate'

For the purpose of this study, continuity was defined as follows:

$$\text{Continuity} = \frac{\text{counts at day } d,\ t}{\text{theoretical number of counts}}$$

Where d ranged from 1–69 days, from the 32nd to the 42nd gestational week, and t was the time (morning, afternoon or evening) when the count was carried out.

Computation of daily fetal movement record

Sadovsky and colleagues[4] recommended the extrapolation of the number of counted movements to a 12-hour period to obtain the daily fetal movement record (DFMR). The following formula was used:

$$\text{DFMR} = \frac{\text{count} \times 720\ \text{min}}{\text{time during which the mother is instructed to count (min)}}$$

where the count is the mean or median number of kicks perceived. When the authors gave a range for duration or counts (e.g. 17–30 in the study by Jarvis and MacDonald[9]), the simple arithmetic mean (e.g. 23.5) was used for computation of DFMR.

Effectiveness of fetal movement counting

Initially, fetal movement counts were introduced by Sadovsky in at-risk pregnancies. Though many followers utilized the technique, few evaluations were made in at-risk pregnancies, as is discussed in the review by Grant and Elbourne[6].

Extension from selective use in a risk population to a policy of systematic counting in unselected pregnancies was then reported, with highly encouraging results in simple experimental designs[10–12]. A randomized trial in Denmark also gave very encouraging results[13]. All of these studies took place in one single clinical setting, leading to small samples and insufficient power. Two large studies did not confirm the potential benefit of routine formal counting in all pregnancies[8,14].

Explanations were sought regarding the discrepancy between the good results of the routine test in small studies and the disappointing results in large multicenter trials. The two most evident were the choice of the count-to-ten regimen and possible difficulties related to acceptability and compliance.

Feasibility and compliance

Data from the Multicenter Fetal Movement Trial (MFMT)

Compliance can be assessed through the 1-month 'in-depth phase' of the trial during which women's charts were collected. Compliance with counting posed problems for the Belgian counting hospitals. The percentage of women who had filled in their charts in the five hospitals randomized to counting were: 15%, 52%, 54%, 60% and 95%. Nor did the hospital where 95% of women were effectively counting achieve this result without effort; in this hospital, charts were collected all through the trial, a monthly assessment was made of the staff from the inception of the trial, and, in the months when the participation rate lowered, active reminding of staff and women was organized. In the other countries taking part in the MFMT study (Ireland, Sweden, the UK and the USA), there was no evidence of such difficulties and the overall rate of counting was 81%.

Data from the French multicenter study

In the French study, two aspects of compliance were addressed: what proportion of women agreed to count, and, among the women who attempted to count, how many continued? Between 42 and 90% of women started counting and continuity was even more disappointing: at best, between 35 and 37 weeks, participation never exceeded 55%. Women were not more likely to count if the recommended time was 30 rather than 60 min. The time of day did not have any impact either.

There were 31 women who wished to stop counting. They were invited to write comments on their charts before returning them. A selection of these statements can be found in Table 1.

Data from the review of the literature

Compliance with counting has been repeatedly evaluated, although it is not always clear for how many consecutive days women were assessed. Results have been summarized in Table 2, where they have been ranked from the highest to the lowest. Compliance seems to be related to the size of the study and the type (nationality, education, motivation) of pregnant population observed, the compliance being better in small studies and in high-risk patients. There is no link between the counting schedule and compliance, although small studies have suggested that the count-to-ten regimen is the most acceptable[15].

Table 1 Translation of comments by French women who decided to stop counting fetal movements

(1) 'It is very difficult to count the baby's kicks. They are habitual and one expects them to occur. To count, one has to concentrate and interrupt all other activity'

(2) 'It moves all day'

(3) 'I have a daughter of two and a half, and I can't find time to concentrate to count the baby's kicks; to count I would have to do nothing else'

(4) 'The baby never moved at the same hour, and I never managed to count because I didn't have time'

(5) 'I did not count, because I am anxious by nature, and I worried when the count decreased'

(6) 'I did not count because I got the impression that when I started counting, I could no longer feel the movements'

(7) 'I cannot see any benefit to counting'

Table 2 Women's compliance in published studies

Year	*Author*	*Country of study*	*Method of Count*	*Population*	*Compliance*
1986	Draper *et al*[22]	UK	count to 10	All	124/127 (98%)
1989	Moore and Piacquiadio[12]	California, USA	count to 10	Military	256/273 (94%)
1994	Liston *et al*[35]	USA	NA	All, RCT	552/613 (90%)
1989	Grant *et al*[8]	UK, Ireland, Sweden	count to 10	All‡	NA (81%)
1981	Harper *et al*[30]	New York, USA	3 × 60 min*	High-risk	77/96 (80%)
1983	Neldam[31]	Denmark	3 × 60 min†	All, RCT	1181/1562 (76%)
1984	Valentin *et al*[32]	Sweden	15 min (pm)	All	1300/1914 (68%)
1979	Henrion and Heard[19]	Paris, France	3 × 30 min	High-risk	200/285 (70%)
1981	Benhamou and Tournaire[18]	Paris, France	3 × 20 min	High-risk	169/288 (59%)
1985	Thompson and Wheeler[33]	UK	count to 10	All	46/83 (55%)
1992	Alexander[34]	Lille, France	3 × 30 min	All	530/1100 (48%)

*Three times a day (morning, afternoon and evening); †three days in each week; ‡in-depth phase (UK, Ireland and Sweden's participation in randomized controlled trial); RCT, randomized controlled trial; NA, not available

Optimal counting schedule and daily fetal movement record

Data from the French multicenter study

It had been assumed that the number of kicks perceived per hour would be roughly double the number of kicks per half hour. This turned out to be a gross misjudgement. Table 3 shows that median counts in 30 min and 60 min were never significantly different. This unexpected observation also holds true for the lower centiles of the distribution. These lower centiles constitute the thresholds for alarm and reporting.

This lack of difference between the absolute number of counts at 30 and 60 min holds true whatever the gestational age, even close to term when the number of kicks has decreased. It is also independent of the time of day (morning, afternoon or evening), which is taken into consideration.

Table 3 Centiles for evening count (30 or 60 min) from the French multicenter study

Gestational week	*Duration of count (min)*	*n*	*Centile* 5%	10%	15%	50%	90%	95%
32	30	39	5	6	9	25	115	136
	60	132	4	6	7	21	71	100
33	30	52	4	6	7	27	70	90
	60	190	4	6	7	19	71	94
34	30	66	3	5	7	21	71	97
	60	218	3	5	6	16	68	91
35	30	64	3	4	6	18	55	79
	60	233	3	4	6	16	65	84
36	30	69	3	5	6	20	61	83
	60	215	3	4	5	14	57	78
37	30	70	4	6	8	18	51	69
	60	206	3	4	5	16	60	91
38	30	52	4	5	6	16	47	69
	60	171	2	3	5	16	57	65
39	30	36	4	5	5	15	32	42
	60	106	2	3	4	14	56	67

Data from the review of the literature

Similar conclusions can be drawn from the analysis of published data. A very large variation in the instructions given to women was noted: the extremes for duration of count ranged from 10 min[16] to 12 h[17]. This observation has led us to challenge the meaning of Sadovski's DFMR, in which an extrapolation is made of the movements counted during the counting period to what they would have been if counting had been continued over 24 h. Such a computation is presented in Table 4 for data in the literature which were presented as a mean: DFMR would then vary between 96 and 2160 kicks per day, according to the population, a 20-fold difference! Similar observations can be made for the papers where results are presented as a median and for fixed-count schemes (count-to-ten adaptations).

Discussion

Because the intervention has not proved to be effective in unselected pregnancies, the only discussion possible pertains to recommendations in situations of medium risk or low technology, or when the women spontaneously report decreased activity. This is

Table 4 Review of the literature and computation of the daily fetal movement record (DFMR): fixed-time count – mean kicks in 12 h

Year	*Author*	*Population*	*No. of patients in study*	*Duration of count (min)*	*Count**	*DFMR (mean computation)*
1977	Spellacy *et al.*[16]	LR	37	10	10–50	2160
1978	Gettinger *et al.*[36]	LR	40	45	31	496
1979	Jarvis and MacDonald[9]	LR	35	180	17–30	96
1979	Hertogs *et al.*[37]	LR	20	30	0–50	600
1980	Birkenfeld *et al.*[38]	R	36	90	18–22	160
1981	Harper *et al.*[30]	Mixed	91	180	NA	212
1981	Weinstein *et al.*[39]	Mixed	50	90	36	288
1981	Weinstein *et al.*[39]	Mixed	50	20	15.4	554
1981	Benhamou and Tournaire[18]	R	91	20	NA	1029
1982	Rayburn[40]	NA	NA	60	20–32	312
1986	Aboulafia *et al.*[41]	LR	NA	90	NA	350
1987	Swartjes and van Geijn[42]	LR	186	120	28–35	189
1987	Kindt *et al.*[43]	NA	30	30	12.5	300

*Number of kicks in minutes of count (values reported in original paper); LR, low-risk; R, at-risk; NA, not available

the case in post-term pregnancy, mild pre-eclampsia, adequately controlled insulin-dependent diabetes, etc. We would suggest that, in such cases and if daily surveillance with more sophisticated technology is not being used, fetal movement counts may well be a useful adjunct to weekly or even bi-weekly heart traces. We are aware that a sufficiently large randomized trial would be necessary to validate this assertion. In the meantime, we would suggest using the simplest and shortest technique: probably count in the evening, after a meal, and count either to ten or for 30 min, whichever is finished first. The validity of fetal movement counting may well vary quite widely from one country to another. There is a culture aspect: in the French study, there were negative comments concerning the method from the mothers (Table 1); furthermore, French caregivers have also expressed their reluctance, both in the study ['difficile de les inciter à compter' (difficult to get them to count)] and in the published data ['une étude astreignante et fastidieuse'[18] (an exacting and tedious study); 'il est indespensable que la femme accepte la méthode sans réserve'[19] (it is essential that the woman accepts the method without reserve)]. Biological variations in fetal activity or maternal perceptivity can be hypothesized. Population differences in fetal biophysical and behavioral characteristics have been reported between Asian, black and white neonates[20]. Even though such differences are confirmed by further studies, it remains to be seen whether they have any impact on maternal perception. It is more likely that compliance with counting is largely behavioral. The capacity to count is not influenced by intellectual or social conditions[21]. On the other hand, two studies have shown the psychological effect of counting. In the first[22], in the UK, results were equivocal, with 55% satisfied and 49% worried out of 132 women. In the second study[5], bonding was enhanced in 213 counting women when compared to controls.

Practices of self-care in pregnancy may be strongly dependent on the organization of health care. They may be more prevalent in countries where costs are powerfully contained, either by free-market forces or by a centralized national health system. In this context, French women are probably less familiar with self-care techniques.

Only assumptions can be made concerning the mechanism of the effect of duration of count on the amount of kicks perceived. Two explanations are offered: one mechanism is that women's threshold of attention to fetal movements decreases with time. This is a well-known phenomenon for most repetitive tasks. A second explanation may be that women do not start their counts on a random basis, but are more likely to start counting precisely at the moment when they are reminded to count by a set of kicks.

BIOPHYSICAL PROFILE, VIBROACOUSTIC STIMULATION AND FETAL BEHAVIOR

These three techniques rely on technology, most often ultrasound and/or cardiotocography and sometimes Doppler.

Materials and methods

A general review of the literature was performed. This review did not aim to be complete, except with regard to randomized trials and blind elaboration of characteristics of the test.

The biophysical profile

The biophysical profile, sometimes referred to as Manning's score was first described in the 1980s[23]; it has sometimes been compared to a fetal Apgar score. It uses five criteria, each scored 0–2, leading to a total of 10/10 in the best possible case and 0/10 in the worst. Of the five criteria, four are assessed with ultrasound: fetal movements, fetal tone, fetal breathing movements and amniotic fluid volume, while fetal heart rate is assessed by electronic monitoring.

Fetal biophysical profile assessment requires equipment (an ultrasound machine and a cardiotocograph) and is time consuming. It has always been restricted to compromised or at-risk pregnancies. Its main use is to aid the decision to continue or interrupt pregnancy in the presence of fetal compromise. Fetal biophysical profile takes, on average, 20 min to perform and this may be one reason why it has not gained wide popularity in parts of the world, such as Belgium. Belgium functions on listed 'fee-for-act' payment schemes, and whilst a fetal biophysical profile cannot be billed, a Doppler takes up less time and can be billed.

A Cochrane overview was performed by Alfirevic and Neilson[24] on three out of the four randomized trials published before 1995. It was found that, 15 years after the introduction of the test and after reports of observational studies on tens of thousands of pregnancies, less than 3000 women had been enrolled into randomized trials; furthermore, at this point, the available data are not sufficient to reach any definite conclusion about the benefit or otherwise of the biophysical profile as a test of fetal well-being in compromised pregnancies. No new randomized trial was identified for 1998 or 1999.

Outside the randomized trial paradigm, the fetal biophysical profile seems very promising. Various studies have shown a good predictive value[25], the main problem being that the test has never been used blind. Using the ecological approach, Manning and colleagues[23], in a recent population-based study on cerebral palsy, found that antepartum assessment by fetal biophysical profile scoring was associated with a significant reduction in the incidence of cerebral palsy compared with untested patients.

Most reviews of methods of assessment of the compromised fetus suggest that the two best are Doppler and fetal biophysical profile. They may well be complementary, as fetal activity may be a better reflection of the neurological state of the fetus, while Doppler reflects circulatory physiology. Such suggestions are only conjectural at this point and, as had been said earlier, a large trial in compromised fetuses should be performed in centers where the fetal biophysical profile is not in use at present.

Vibroacoustic stimulation

Vibroacoustic stimulation is a technique which assesses the fetal reaction to vibroacoustic stimulation. This reaction may be assessed through cardiotocography[26], Doppler[27] or the assessment of fetal movements by ultrasound or by the mother.

In a review paper, Smith[28] concluded that the technique is safe, but that further research is needed to characterize the optimal frequency, duration, intensity and choice of stimulus to provide consistent responses. The literature presents a confusing array of studies using different methods, which makes comparison of results among institutions and investigators difficult. Vibroacoustic stimulation appears to be a reasonable and safe clinical technique. Additional prospective investigation is necessary to characterize further how this technique can be more useful clinically.

Fetal behavior

Fetal behavior studies are not usually considered to be tests of well-being, but rather contributions to the understanding of fetal physiology. A wide array of behaviors has been described: sleep cycle, yawning, hiccups, thumb sucking, startle movements, right-handedness, etc. In addition, the effect of external parameters (meals, caffeine, sugar, hyperventilation, maternal exercise, various medications) on these behaviors has also been broadly studied. At present, there is no use for the assessment of fetal behavior as a test of fetal well-being. Nevertheless, there are suggestions that fetal behavior may adequately predict later childhood behavior, such as crying[29]. Any tool which has good predictive power may well end up as a test of fetal well-being.

GENERAL CONCLUSION

None of the techniques that we have discussed here can at present be promoted as 'evidence-based medicine'. In low-risk pregnancies, routine fetal movement counts have been tested in a randomized trial and did not prove to be effective. In at-risk pregnancies, each of the four techniques presents theoretical advantages, which were discussed above, but none of them has been appropriately evaluated. As long as this is the case, the techniques will continue to be used in some centers, but cannot be promoted as effective modes of surveillance of the jeopardized fetus. To this day, the only test of fetal well-being that has been evaluated and proved to be effective is Doppler.

ACKNOWLEDGEMENT

The MFMT-F research project was supported by the Institut National de la Santé et de la Recherche Médicale (France) (research grant RG/SR/no. 595).

REFERENCES

1. Thompson D, ed. *The Concise Oxford English Dictionary*, 9th edn. Oxford: Clarendon Press, 1995
2. Playfair WS. *A Treatise on the Science and Practice of Midwifery*, vol II, 5th edn. London: Smith Elder, 1884
3. Mathews DD. Foetal movements and foetal well-being. *Lancet* 1973;1:1315
4. Sadovsky E, Polishuk WZ, Mahler Y. Correlation between electromagnetic recording and maternal assessment of foetal movement. *Lancet* 1973;1:1141–3
5. Mikhail MS, Freda MC, Merkatz RB, Polizzotto R, Mazloom E, Merkatz IR. The effect of fetal movement counting on maternal attachment to fetus. *Am J Obstet Gynecol* 1991;165:988–91
6. Grant A, Elbourne D. Foetal movement counting as a test of foetal well-being. In Chalmers I, *et al.*, eds. *Effective care in Pregnancy and Childbirth*. Oxford: Oxford University Press, 1989:440–54
7. Baskett TF, Liston RM. Foetal movement monitoring: clinical application. *Clin Perinatol* 1989;16:613–25
8. Grant A, Elbourne D, Valentin L, Alexander S. Routine formal foetal movement counting and risk of antepartum late death in normally formed singletons. *Lancet* 1989;2:345–9
9. Jarvis GJ, MacDonald HN. Foetal movements in small-for-dates babies. *Br J Obstet Gynaecol* 1979;86:724–7
10. Westgate J, Jamieson M. Stillbirths and foetal movements. *NZ Med J* 1986;99:114–16
11. Boog G. Le comptage des mouvements foetaux. Une méthode simple et sûre de surveillance de la grossesse. Cervix and prediction of preterm birth. *Rev Fr Gynécol Obstét* 1988;83:693–5
12. Moore T, Piacquiadio K. A prospective evaluation of fetal movement screening to reduce the incidence of antepartum fetal death. *Am J Obstet Gynecol* 1989;96:298–307

13. Neldam S. Foetal movements as an indicator of foetal well-being. *Lancet* 1980;1:1222–4
14. Lobb MO, Beazley JM, Haddad NG. A controlled study of daily foetal movement counts in the prevention of stillbirths. *J Obstet Gynaecol* 1985;6:87–91
15. Smith CV, Davis SA, Rayburn WF. Patients' acceptance of monitoring foetal movement. A randomised comparison of charting techniques. *J Reprod Med* 1992;37:144–6
16. Pearson JF, Weaver JB. Foetal activity and foetal well-being: an evaluation. *Br Med J* 1976;1:1305–7
17. Spellacy WN, Cruz AC, Gelman SR, Buhi WC. Fetal movements and placental lactogen levels for fetal–placental evaluation. *Obstet Gynecol* 1977;49:113–15
18. Benhamou M, Tournaire M. Le compte des mouvements actifs du fetus. *J Gynecol Obstet Biol Reprod* 1981;10:449–58
19. Henrion R, Heard I. Surveillance du fœtus *in utero* grâce au compte des mouvements actifs. *Nouv Presse Méd* 1979;8:3113–15
20. Johnson TR, Paine LL, Strobino DM, Witter FR. Population differences affect the results of fetal non stress test results. *Am J Obstet Gynecol* 1998;179:779–83
21. Leader LR, Baillie P, van Schalkwyk DB. Fetal movements and fetal outcome: a prospective study. *Obstet Gynecol* 1981:57:431–6
22. Draper J, Field S, Thomas H, Hare MJ. Women's views on keeping fœtal movement charts. *Br J Obstet Gynaecol* 1986;93:334–8
23. Manning FA, Bondaji N, Harman CR, *et al.* Fetal assessment based on fetal biophysical profile scoring. VIII. The incidence of cerebral palsy in tested and untested perinates. *Am J Obstet Gynecol* 1998;178:696–706
24. Alfirevic Z, Neilson JP. Biophysical profile for fœtal assessment in high risk pregnancies [Cochrane Review]. In *The Cochrane Library*, Issue 4. Oxford: Update Software, 1998
25. Miller DA, Rabello YA, Paul RH. The modified biophysical profile: antepartum testing in the 1990s. *Am J Obstet Gynecol* 1996;174:812–17
26. Bartnicki J, Dimer JA, Hertwig K, Dudenhausen JW. Computerised cardiotocography following vibroacoustic stimulation of premature fetuses. *Gynecol Obstet Invest* 1998;45: 73–6
27. Loy GL, Lin CC, Chien EK, Kim JH, Chiang LM. Cerebral and umbilical vascular resistance response to vibroacoustic stimulation in growth-restricted fetuses. *Obstet Gynecol* 1997;90:947–52
28. Smith CV. Vibroacoustic stimulation. *Clin Obstet Gynecol* 1995;38:68–77
29. St James-Roberts I, Menon Johansson P. Predicting infant cry from fœtal movement data: an exploratory study. *Early Hum Dev* 1999;54:55–62
30. Harper RG, Greenberg M, Farahani G, Glassman I, Kierney CM. Fetal movement, biochemical and biophysical parameters, and the outcome of pregnancy. *Am J Obstet Gynecol* 1981;141:39–42
31. Neldam S. Fetal movements as an indicator of fetal well-being. *Dan Med Bull* 1983;30: 274–80
32. Valentin L, Lofgren O, Marsal K, Gullberg B. Subjective recording of fetal movements. III. Screening of a pregnant population; the clinical significance of decreased fetal movement counts. *Acta Obstet Gynecol Scand* 1984;65:753–8

33. Thompson SL, Wheeler T. Compliance and maternal fetal movement counting [Letter]. *Lancet* 1985;2:1122
34. Alexander S. Etude multicentrique française du compte des mouvements fœtaux – MFMT-F. Lille/Bruxelles: rapport à la direction générale de l'INSERM, 1992
35. Liston RM, Bloom K, Zimmer P. The psychological effects of counting foetal movements. *Birth* 1994;21:35–40
36. Gettinger A, Roberts AB, Campbell S. Comparison between subjective and ultrasound assessments of fetal movement. *Br Med J* 1978;2:88–9
37. Hertogs K, Roberts AB, Cooper D, Griffin DR, Campbell S. Maternal perception of fetal motor activity. *Br Med J* 1979;2:1183–5
38. Birkenfeld A, Laufer N, Sadovsky E. Diurnal variation of fetal activity. *Obstet Gynecol* 1980;55:417–19
39. Weinstein D, Navot D, Sadovsky E. Antepartum ultrasound foetal heart rate monitoring and foetal movements. *J Obstet Gynaecol* 1981;2:85–7
40. Rayburn WF. Antepartum foetal assessment: foetal activity monitoring. *Clin Perinatol* 1982;9:231–52
41. Aboulafia Y, Sadovsky E, Simon A, Ohel G, Zajicek G. Fetal activity in pregnancies complicated by lupus erythematosus. *Arch Gynecol* 1986;237:181–5
42. Swartjes JM, van Geijn HP. Maternal perception of fetal movements: the optimal duration of a recording period. *Eur J Gynecol Reprod Biol* 1987;25:97–103
43. Kindt von J, Erhardt U, Retzke U, Stübe G. Subjektives registrieren der Kindsbewegungen. Abhängigkeit von typologisch-psychischen Merkmalen der Schwangeren. *Zent Gynäkol* 1987;109:1527-31

Urogynaecology

3

Cesarean section to prevent female incontinence

J. M. van Geelen

INTRODUCTION

Urinary incontinence is a common and distressing problem for many women. A recent meta-analysis of epidemiological studies published in the English literature which looked at the prevalence of urinary incontinence in community-dwelling populations concluded that 'a 30% prevalence of any urine loss during a 12-month period is a plausible estimate'[1]. Although not life-threatening, incontinence may considerably influence the quality of life for those affected and has significant cost implications for health services.

Child-bearing has always been associated with the onset of urinary incontinence, but the precise role of pregnancy and delivery in the development of persistent stress incontinence remains unclear. During the last two decades, basic research and clinical studies have provided new insights into the pathogenesis of this condition.

This review comprehensively looks at our present knowledge of the effects of pregnancy and childbirth on the mechanisms of continence.

EPIDEMIOLOGY

Urinary incontinence has long been considered a common sequel to labor. Francis[2] was the first to carry out a prospective study on 400 healthy women. She observed that 53% of primigravid women and 85% of multigravid women experienced stress incontinence to some degree during pregnancy. Persistent incontinence after childbirth was observed in 6% of the women. She concluded that 'stress incontinence rarely, if ever, appears for the first time after childbirth if it had not occurred before or during the pregnancy'[2]. Figures reported by other investigators in subsequent studies are at variance with these findings (Table 1)[3–8]. These discrepancies may be due to differences in definition, and variations in question techniques and observation period. In spite of the differences in incidence figures, all epidemiological data indicate a high incidence of urinary incontinence during pregnancy. In a smaller percentage (5–10%) of women, urinary incontinence persists after childbirth or arises *de novo* in the puerperium. Of the women who were delivered by Cesarean section, none continued to have stress incontinence after childbirth. However, the protective effect of Cesarean section is limited, as the prevalence of urinary incontinence in women with three or more Cesarean sections is similar to that in women delivering vaginally[9].

PREGNANCY AND URINARY INCONTINENCE

Francis[2] carried out lateral urethrocystography in late pregnancy in women with stress incontinence and normal healthy controls. She observed the radiological sign of an 'absent posterior urethrovesical angle' as a striking feature in patients with stress

Table 1 The onset of stress incontinence

	During pregnancy (%)	*Persistent after childbirth* (%)	*De novo after childbirth* (%)
Francis (1960)[2]** (n = 400)	67	6	—
Beck and Hsu (1965)[3] (n = 1000)	20	10	4.4
Stanton *et al.* (1980)[4] (n = 83 primigravid women)	39	6	—
(n = 98 multigravid women)	42	11	—
Iosif (1981)[5] (n = 1411)	16	5	4
van Geelen *et al.* (1982)[6]** (n = 42)*	24	5	2.4
Dimpfl *et al.* (1992)[7]** (n = 290)	53	8	3.7
Viktrup *et al.* (1992)[8]**	32	19	7
(n = 305)*	1	2	1 (ICS)

*Primigravid women only; **Cesarean sections taken into account; ICS, International Continence Society incontinence, whereas in continent pregnant controls, the anatomy of the posterior urethrovesical angle was unaltered. Loss of the posterior urethrovesical angle is often associated with stress incontinence, but is not considered a diagnostic symptom as it may be present in many women with perfect bladder control.

Studies carrying out simultaneous urethrocystometry and urethral pressure profilometry during pregnancy and after childbirth have shown that, in healthy continent women, the variables of the urethral sphincter mechanism at rest and during coughing hardly change during the course of pregnancy[6,10]. In the women who developed stress incontinence of some kind during the pregnancy under observation, values of the urethral pressure profile variables were below the median values for the study population. In addition, defective transmission of intra-abdominal pressure to the urethra, resulting in a decreased urethral closure pressure during stress, could be observed. The results of these studies lead one to conclude that stress incontinence manifests itself in those women who have a lower urethral resistance and defective transmission of intra-abdominal pressure over the urethra early in pregnancy when compared with continent controls. These observations confirm the earlier suggestion by Francis[2] that an inherent weakness of the urethral closure mechanism and periurethral supportive tissue is the underlying basis for the development of stress incontinence. In an elegant study carried out in 1990, Landon and colleagues demonstrated that, during pregnancy, the mechanical properties of fascia tissue alter[11]. Pregnancy was associated with a significant reduction in collagen stiffness when compared with non-pregnant controls. Pregnant fascia is more elastic, but also much weaker, than non-pregnant fascia. Much less stress is required to produce tissue failure and therefore the tensile strength of the fascia is reduced. These changes most probably represent necessary physiological accommodation during pregnancy, but reduced tensile strength implies that pregnant fascia is more easily irreversibly damaged or ruptured.

In 1998, Falconer and associates[12] from Sweden were able to identify differences in the organization of collagen fibrils between stress incontinent women and healthy controls of the same age. Their major findings were a significantly higher collagen concentration in combination with higher cross-linking in women with genuine stress incontinence. These biochemical changes were accompanied by ultrastructural differences in the form of a significantly larger collagen fibril diameter. An increase in collagen concentration and simultaneously increased cross-linking affect the tensile strength of the connective tissue. These observations suggest that a constitutional or genetic disorder underlies the onset of stress incontinence.

During pregnancy, the growth of the uterus together with hormonal changes will affect the mechanical properties of the connective tissue and will give rise to incontinence in those women who are predisposed due to defective connective tissue. In many women, these tissue changes will be reversible. In some women, however, the dimensions of tissue stretch lead to tissue failure and persistent incontinence after childbirth.

VAGINAL DELIVERY AND INCONTINENCE

Anatomical aspects

At the onset of labor, the position of the bladder base and the urethrovesical junction are at the level of a line joining the lower border of the symphysis pubis and the tip of the sacrum. With the progress of labor, the bladder neck and the proximal urethra are displaced forward. The bladder base is rolled up forwards from behind and comes into line with the urethra, giving the impression that the urethra becomes elongated. Rotation of the bladder base from its normal horizontal position to a vertical position stretches its fascial investment between the bladder and vagina[13,14]. The extent of this stretching depends upon the relationship between the fetal size and pelvic capacity. Some trauma is incurred by the bladder and urethra during labor and during a vaginal delivery. The extent of the traumatic changes varies from increased edema and mucosal congestion to varying degrees of submucosal hemorrhage and sometimes actual capillary oozing. These findings are most marked in the region of the bladder neck, trigone and around the ureteral orifices. Within a few hours after delivery, the urethrovesical junction and the bladder base resume their normal shape and revert to their proper position, as seen in the non-pregnant state. The traumatic changes in the bladder wall tend to disappear during the first few days after childbirth.

Dynamic aspects

After vaginal delivery, mean values of urethral sphinter function (i.e. urethral closure pressure and functional urethral length) are significantly decreased when compared with values at 8 weeks' amenorrhea or with values in healthy nulliparous women[6,10]. In addition, the amplitude of vascular pulsations in the urethral wall in the postpartum recordings was notably decreased in almost all women delivered vaginally. In the women who were delivered by elective Cesarean section, no such changes could be observed. In a retrospective study comparing continent women with incontinent women, carried out in order to investigate the effect of childbirth on the subsequent integrity of the urethral sphincter mechanism, Tapp and co-workers[15] found by urethral profilometry that vaginal delivery mainly affects the distal part of the urethral sphincter mechanism. These authors found no significant correlation between birth weight and changes in urethral pressure variables or between birth weight and pressure transmission ratios.

Other investigators examined the relationship of the mode of delivery and other obstetric factors with the prevalence of incontinence after childbirth[6–9]. The incidence of incontinence increased with increasing parity, with a significant increase after the fourth delivery[9]. The mode of delivery (i.e. spontaneous versus instrumental vaginal delivery) and obstetric factors, such as birth weight, head circumference, length of second stage of labor, and presence or absence of an episiotomy, do not seem to affect the incidence of stress incontinence after delivery. In women having epidural anesthesia during labor, the incidence of postpartum stress incontinence was significantly lower than in those without regional anesthesia during delivery[7].

Neurogenic aspects

Over the last decade, a few studies have investigated the effect of childbirth on the pelvic floor by carrying out pudendal nerve function tests[16–18]. Vaginal delivery causes pudendal nerve damage in 80% of women delivering their first baby. In women delivered by elective Cesarean section, no denervation was observed, whereas in women who had a Cesarean section during labor, denervation damage was present. These findings indicate that labor itself is important in the denervation damage sustained during childbirth. In most women, pudendal nerve damage causes few or no clinical symptoms. In a few, denervation is severe and associated with incontinence. Except for a long active second stage of labor, other obstetric factors do not significantly influence the degree of denervation[17].

Delivery and anal incontinence

Overt sphincter damage due to a third- or fourth-degree tear occurs in approximately 0.5–1% of women during vaginal delivery in centers where mediolateral episiotomy is practiced. The incidence and importance of occult anal sphincter damage during routine vaginal delivery are unknown. Sultan and associates[19] carried out a prospective clinical study on 150 pregnant women 6 weeks before delivery and 6 weeks after childbirth, using anal endosonography, manometry, measurement of pudendal nerve terminal motor latency and perineometry. Their results showed that, in 35% of primiparous and 44% of multiparous women, occult sphincter defect could be demonstrated. All these defects occurred in the anterior portion of the anal sphincter. In women undergoing elective Cesarean section, no sphincter defects could be observed. The defect persisted in all women studied again at 6 months. About one-third of the women with a sphincter defect developed bowel symptoms: fecal urgency and/or incontinence. The authors concluded that vaginal delivery, especially the first vaginal delivery, causes mechanical trauma to the anal sphincter and injury to the pudendal nerve leading to bowel symptoms in about 10% of women. These results show a surprisingly high incidence and necessitate long-term follow-up. Women with a sphincter defect carry a greater risk of aggravation of their problems after subsequent vaginal delivery.

CONCLUSION

In conclusion, stress incontinence as a symptom is a common feature during pregnancy, reflecting an inherent or constitutional weakness of the supportive pelvic structures. In the majority of women, symptoms will resolve completely in the immediate post-partum period. However, in 5–10% of the women with stress incontinence during pregnancy, symptoms will persist, leading to occasional incontinence during stress. Only in a minority of women can the onset of symptoms be attributed to vaginal delivery itself. Symptoms recur with each subsequent pregnancy and become progressively worse, so that in the long term the woman is left with objectively demonstrable incontinence. Consequently, there is a linear relationship between the number of childbirths and the risk of developing incontinence. None of the women delivered by elective Cesarean section continued to have or developed stress incontinence in the puerperium. However, the protective effect of Cesarean section is limited, as, after three or more Cesarean sections, the prevalence of incontinence is similar to that in women delivered vaginally. In addition, there are no indications that Cesarean section is protective against stress incontinence later in life[20].

REFERENCES

1. Herzog AR, Fultz NH. Prevalence and incidence of urinary incontinence in community-dwelling populations. *J Am Geriatr Soc* 1990;38:2732–81
2. Francis WJA. The onset of stress incontinence. *J Obstet Gynaecol Br Commonw* 1960;67:899–903
3. Beck PP, Hsu N. Pregnancy, childbirth and the menopause related to the development of stress incontinence. *Am J Obstet Gynecol* 1965;91:820–3
4. Stanton SL, Kerr-Wilson R, Grant-Harris V. The incidence of urological symptoms in normal pregnancy. *Br J Obstet Gynaecol* 1980;87:897–900
5. Iosif S. Stress incontinence during pregnancy and in puerperium. *Int J Gynaecol Obstet* 1981;19:13–20
6. van Geelen JM, Lemmens WAJG, Eskes TKAB, *et al.* The urethral pressure profile in pregnancy and after delivery in healthy nulliparous women. *Am J Obstet Gynecol* 1982;144:636–49
7. Dimpfl T, Hesse U, Schüssler B. Incidence and cause of post partum urinary stress incontinence. *Eur J Obstet Gynecol Reprod Biol* 1992;43:29–33
8. Viktrup L, Lose G, Rollf M, *et al.* The symptom of stress incontinence caused by pregnancy or delivery in primiparas. *Obstet Gynecol* 1992;79:945–9
9. Wilson PD, Herbison RM, Herbison GB. Obstetric practice and the prevalence of urinary incontinence three months after delivery. *Br J Obstet Gynaecol* 1996;103:154–61

10. Iosif S, Ulmsten U. Comparative urodynamic studies of continent and stress incontinent women in pregnancy and in the puerperium. *Am J Obstet Gynecol* 1981;140:645–50
11. Landon CR, Crofts CE, Smith ARB, *et al.* Mechanical properties of fascia during pregnancy: a possible factor in the development of stress incontinence of urine. *Contemp Rev Obstet Gynecol* 1990;2:40–6
12. Falconer C, Blomgren B, Johansson O, *et al.* Different organization of collagen fibrils in stress incontinent women of fertile age. *Acta Obstet Gynaecol Scand* 1998;77:87–94
13. Kantor HI, Miller JE, Dunlap JC. The urinary bladder during labor. *Am J Obstet Gynecol* 1949;58:354–64
14. Malpas P, Jeffcoate TNA, Lister UM. The displacement of the bladder and urethra during labor. *J Obstet Gynaecol Br Emp* 1949;56:949–60
15. Tapp A, Cardozo L, Versi E, *et al.* The effect of vaginal delivery on the urethral sphincter. *Br J Obstet Gynaecol* 1998;95:142–6
16. Snooks SJ, Swash M, Setchell M, *et al.* Injury to the innervation of pelvic floor sphincter musculature in childbirth. *Lancet* 1984;36:546–56
17. Allen RE, Hosker GL, Smith ARB, *et al.* Pelvic floor damage and childbirth: a neurophysiologic study. *Br J Obstet Gynaecol* 1990;97:770–9
18. Tetzschner T, Sörensen M, Lose G, *et al.* Pudendal nerve function during pregnancy and after delivery. *Int Urogynecol J* 1997;8:66–8
19. Sultan AH, Kamm MA, Hudson CN, *et al.* Anal sphincter disruption during vaginal delivery. *N Engl J Med* 1993;329:1905–11
20. Gordon H, Logue M. Perineal muscle function after childbirth. *Lancet* 1985;2:123–5

4

Micro-invasive surgical techniques for the treatment of urogynaecological disorders: traditional procedures

E. Petri

INTRODUCTION

A myriad of surgical procedures has been described for the treatment of urinary stress incontinence. Taking into account all different techniques, modifications and submodifications, more than 200 procedures can be found in the literature. For decades, the aim of the gynecological surgeon has been to reconstruct a damaged pelvic floor, disregarding functional aspects; in contrast, urologists disregarded the anatomy and wanted to restore nothing but function in their operations. Both were wrong!

Burch's colposuspension and its modifications have been the 'gold standard' of treatment for the last 20 years, and have been accepted in both specialties. Since the early 1990s, endoscopists have been looking for new ways forward with their fascinating laparoscopic approaches. It took urogynecologists nearly a decade just to accept the possibilities of new micro-invasive approaches; at the same time, traditional operations were modified to involve less invasive surgery, reducing incisions and separation of tissues to a minimum, or using new instruments which allow out-patient operations with local anesthesia tension-free vaginal tape (TVT).

SURGICAL CONCEPTS

The surgical approaches for treatment of sphincter incompetence are different around the world, and are mainly influenced by the medical facilities and resources available. There is a great lack of honesty when a procedure is selected because of 'good experience', 'good outcome' and 'no complications'. We have to accept that health-care systems are different and sometimes do not allow certain operations because the patient cannot afford them. Long-term follow-up with objective and subjective parameters and the acceptance of these data would markedly reduce the number of procedures available. Why is an 'improved' patient counted together with a cured one? What is the definition of 'improved'? The use of 12 pads before and eight after surgery? Who asks elderly patients about sexual intercourse and obstructive micturition, and who asks these questions to a young, hard-working patient after abdominal procedures for abdominal pain?

More than 50% (in some countries more than 75%) of gynecologists still perform vaginal repairs (whatever is meant by and performed using this technique) for the primary treatment of urinary incontinence; similar numbers of needle suspensions are performed by urologists, even though during recent meetings of the American Urological Association and the European Society of Urology (Barcelona, March 1998) there were clear data against using these techniques as good primary procedures.

There are two pathophysiological concepts for the approach:

(1) Repositioning the bladder neck and the proximal urethra back into the abdomino-pelvic pressure transmission zone (e.g. colposuspension and slings);

(2) Re-fixation of the mid-urethra at the place of the maximal urethral closure pressure and the pressure transmission zone, aiming at a replacement of the torn pubo-urethral ligaments (TVT).

GOLD STANDARD

Even though in many European countries the tradition of vaginal repairs together with hysterectomy is surviving and is the treatment of choice with 50–85% of gynecologists, and needle suspension, in spite of unfavorable long-term data world-wide, is the first-choice treatment for many urologists, Burch's colposuspension and its modifications have been looked upon as the 'gold standard' of treatment around the world. Sling procedures experience ups and downs, and use different alloplastic and autologous materials, but are still accepted as the treatment of choice in hypotonic urethra (intrinsic sphincter deficiency) and recurrent severe incontinence. They are now experiencing a revival in American urology.

Burch's colposuspension[1,2], modified by Cowan and Morgan[3] and others, has emerged to give good long-term results subjectively and objectively in follow-ups of up to 20 years, with success rates of 70–80% for primary incontinence and 60–70% for recurrences[4–7]. The most important result from controlled studies in recent years has been the fact that the treatment of recurrences has been up to 20% less effective because of scar tissue formation and partial destruction of neuromuscular structures in the periurethral region. Therefore, it has to be remembered, as Hodgkinson[8] stated as early as 1970, that the typical strategy of gynecologists, to try a vaginal approach first and only in cases of recurrence to use an abdominal technique, should be a thing of the past.

In our institution we performed a modified colposuspension in approximately 1800 patients, performing a small 5–6-cm incision 2 cm above the symphysis pubis, and, after complete blunt dissection of the pelvic side walls, placing two lateral tangential sutures with Ethibond (O-strength, MO–6 needle) so that they are very loosely connected to Cooper's ligament without any tension. In a follow-up of up to 12 years, we reached a cure rate of 80–88% in primary cases and of 71% in recurrences. In a detailed follow-up study of subjective data, we learnt that the satisfaction of the patients is decreased by obstructive micturition and, particularly in hard-working women, by pain in the area of fixation ('colposuspension syndrome')[9].

Comparing the recurrence rates of vaginal repairs and needle suspensions with those of controls within a 2-year follow-up, colposuspension is superior to all other techniques in markedly improving the quality of life in over 50% of patients.

In women with intrinsic sphincter deficiency (ISD) (hypotonic urethra – urethral closure pressure $< 20\ cmH_2O$), there are failure rates of up to 50% because of hypocontractility of the urethra. Recognition of this high-risk group is only one of the indications for preoperative urodynamic work-up. The results of this process should influence the selection of procedure and, following selection, the informed consent of the patient should also be obtained.

Until now, recurrences with hypotonic urethra were an indication for fascial slings in our patients, as described previously[10]. We are now changing strategy towards the tension-free vaginal tape, as described by Ulmsten and Petros[11].

THERAPEUTIC STRATEGY

After exhausting all conservative regimens, including estrogen replacement therapy, physiotherapy, cones and electrotherapy, and urodynamic and morphological proof of sphincter incompetence, the aim of surgical therapy is:

(1) Reconstruction of any relevant pelvic floor defect with independent symptoms (e.g. residual urine from a large cystocele, recurrent urinary tract infection), which, in cases with a central defect, is best achieved by vaginal reconstruction;

(2) Repositioning of the bladder neck region back into 'abdomino-pelvic equilibrium'[12], which is best achieved by an abdominal approach, or, in the future, by TVT;

(3) In recurrences and hypotonic urethra (ISD), a sling procedure is to be recommended; in the future, TVT might be an alternative;

(4) With correct preoperative work-up and correct surgical technique, cure rates between 85 and 90% are possible; even in recurrences, cure rates of 65–80% can be achieved.

REFERENCES

1. Burch JC. Urethrovaginal fixation to Cooper's ligament for correction of stress incontinence, cystocele and prolapse. *Am J Obstet Gynecol* 1961;81:281–90
2. Burch JC. Cooper's ligament urethrovesical suspension for stress incontinence. *Am J Obstet Gynecol* 1968;100:764–72
3. Cowan W, Morgan HR. A simplified retropubic urethropaxy in the treatment of primary and recurrent urinary stress incontinence in the female. *Am J Obstet Gynecol* 1979;133:295–9
4. Stanton SL, Williams JE, Ritchie B. The colposuspension operation for urinary incontinence. *Br J Obstet Gynaecol* 1976;83:890–5
5. Stanton SL, Cardozo LD. A comparison of vaginal and suprapubic surgery in the correction of incontinence due to urethral sphincter incompetence. *Br J Urol* 1979;51:497–9
6. Alcalay M, Monga AK, Stanton SL. Burch colposuspension – how long does it cure stress incontinence? *Neurourol Urodyn* 1994;13:495–6
7. Petri E, Eberhard J. Differenzierter Einsatz verschiedener Inkontinenz – und Deszensusoperationen. In Petri E, ed. *Gynäkologische Urologie*, 2nd edn. Stuttgart: Thieme, 1996:237–59
8. Hodgkinson CP. Stress urinary incontinence – 1970. *Am J Obstet Gynecol* 1970;105: 1141–68

9. Petri E. Retropubic cystourethropexies. In Cardozo L, Staskin D, eds. *Textbook of Female Urology and Urogynaecology*. Oxford: Isis Med. Med, 1999:in press
10. Hohenfellner R, Petri E. Sling procedures. In Stanton SL, Tangho E, eds. *Surgery of Female Incontinence*, 2nd edn. Berlin: Springer, 1986:105–13
11. Ulmsten U, Petros P. Intravaginal sling plasty (IVS): an ambulatory surgical procedure for treatment of female urinary incontinence. *Scand J Urol Nephrol* 1995;29:75–82
12. Richter K. Pathologie der Streßinkontinenz und die anatomischen Möglichkeiten ihrer chirurgischen Behandlung. In Petri E, ed. *Gynäkologische Urologie*, 2nd edn. Stuttgart: Thieme, 1996:221–36

Infertility

5

Genetic risks of IVF and ICSI

M. Barata

INTRODUCTION

Little is known about the effect of *in vitro* fertilization techniques on chromosome abnormalities. There may be a relationship between early chromosomal disorders and specific reproductive technologies. Some studies have found no relationship with stimulation regimes[1,2]. However, in another important study, the results suggest that culture conditions and different stimulation protocols may induce chromosomal abnormalities[3].

With regard to intracytoplasmic sperm injection (ICSI), a very important study, including a prospective study analyzing 868 male and female patients prior to planned ICSI treatment suggests that all partners should be routinely karyotyped before ICSI.

IN VITRO FERTILIZATION

From a review of the studies concerning the effect of *in vitro* fertilization (IVF) techniques it is clear that there is a need to unify IVF procedures in order to assess the effects of follicular induction and chromosomal status.

Hormonal stimulation, gamete collection and embryo culture are all parameters which have an impact on oocyte and embryo morphology. In the case of hormonal stimulation, the main difference concerns the use or not of down-regulation protocols.

Many more mosaic embryos were obtained before 1991 compared to later years. Mosaicism was studied in good quality embryos from four different centers by Munné and colleagues[3]. The conclusion is not clear because each center was largely associated with a particular hormonal regime. However, a more balanced arrangement using various stimulation regimes to a greater extent in each center is not possible because gonadotropin stimulation is now used only in patients who do not respond to down-regulation.

With regard to gamete collection and embryo culture various parameters can have an effect. Temperature; aging of gametes; oxygen tension of 20% compared to 5%; exposure to volatile organic compounds; suboptimal pH or heavy metal ions and visible light exposure are some examples.

In conclusion, we can say that IVF babies have similar chromosome abnormality rates when compared to the general population. This is possible in spite of the effects of IVF on chromosome distribution, as most abnormalities produced at the first mitotic division result in death of the embryo.

INTRACYTOPLASMIC SPERM INJECTION

In a prospective study, Meschede and colleagues analyzed the karyotype of 868 male and female patients prior to ICSI. A total of 33 aberrant karyotypes were diagnosed; 24 of the chromosomal abnormalities were found among the women. Low-level mosaicism for numerical sex chromosome anomalies was diagnosed in 20 individuals, and one patient had the triple X karyotype. Given the high rate of abnormal karyotypes among the females, these authors postulated that routine karyotyping should be performed in both partners prior to ICSI.

It is a well-established fact that the rate of metaphases aneuploid for the X chromosome increases with a woman's advancing age[4]. There is no doubt that abnormal karyotypes are more prevalent among infertile men and women enrolled in ICSI programs than in normal control populations. However, it appears as though the risk for a viable pregnancy with a chromosomal abnormality originating from a parent aberration may not be very high even in this population. These chromosomal anomalies arose *de novo*, possibly because of the advanced age of the women or because of an increased rate of sperm chromosome aneuploidy among infertile men[5]. Govaert and colleagues interestingly noticed however, that the risk for a liveborn child with no unbalanced karyotype that arose from a predisposing parental anomaly may be low after ICSI treatment.

REFERENCES

1. Plachot M, Velga A, Montagut J, *et al.* Are clinical and biological IVF parameters correlated with chromosomal disorders in early life: a multi-centric study. *Hum Reprod* 1986;5:627–35
2. Tejada MI, Mendoza R, Cortostegui B, Benito JA. Chromosome studies in human unfertilized oocytes and uncleaved zygotes after treatment with gonadotropin-releasing hormone analogs. *Fertil Steril* 1991;56:874–80
3. Munné C, Magli A, Adler G, *et al.* Treatment-related chromosome abnormalities in human embryos. *Hum Reprod* 1997;12:780–4
4. Surrallés J, Jeppesen O, Morrison H, *et al.* Analysis of loss of inactive X chromosomes in interphase cells. *Am J Hum Genet* 1996;59:1091–6
5. Van Opstal D, Ios FJ, Ramlakhan S, *et al.* Determination of the parent of origin in nine cases of prenatally detected chromosome aberrations found after intracytoplasmic sperm injection. *Hum Reprod* 1997;12:682–6

6

Adverse effects of assisted reproductive technology

J. G. Schenker

INTRODUCTION

Assisted reproduction is a common practice in modern reproductive medicine. Complications are associated with ovulation induction, ovarian hyperstimulation syndrome, the risk of epithelial ovarian tumors and the extracorporeal methods that are used for *in vitro* fertilization–embryo transfer, gamete intra-Fallopian transfer and zygote intra-Fallopian transfer. These complications are associated with laparoscopy, anesthesia, oocyte retrieval and laboratory facilities. Pregnancies resulting from assisted reproduction are more complicated than spontaneous pregnancies.

Assisted reproduction results in higher rates of ectopic, heterotopic and multifetal pregnancies, as well as higher rates of abortions and premature deliveries. Increased rates of perinatal mortality and morbidity result from prematurity, and higher rates of maternal diseases in pregnancy (pre-eclampsia, diabetes mellitus, bleeding, anemia) contribute to fetal intrauterine growth restriction and maternal morbidity. Assisted reproduction practice should therefore be well controlled in view of the potential for complications both before and during pregnancy.

OVARIAN HYPERSTIMULATION SYNDROME

Ovarian hyperstimulation syndrome (OHSS) is a serious complication affecting ovulation induction[1,2]. Its most severe manifestation takes the form of massive ovarian enlargement and multiple cysts, hemoconcentration and third-space accumulation of fluid. Renal failure and oliguria, hypovolemic shock, thromboembolic episodes, adult respiratory distress syndrome (ARDS) and death may complicate the full-blown clinical syndrome. Based on the clinical presentation and laboratory findings, OHSS is divided into three categories (mild, moderate and severe) and into six grades of severity. Ideally, ovarian ovulation induction should stimulate the ovaries only to a desired level of ovulation. However, the narrow therapeutic range of human menopausal gonadotropin (hMG), as well as other ovulation-induction agents and the occasional unpredictable patient response, makes total prevention of OHSS virtually impossible.

Several risk factors have been reported to be associated with OHSS: young age (< 35 years), asthenic habitus, the presence of polycystic ovary syndrome, pregnancy, human chorionic gonadotropin (hCG) supplementation, high serum estradiol (> 2500 pg/ml), multiple follicles and ultrasonographic ovarian 'necklace sign'[3].

Although the pathophysiology of OHSS has not been completely elucidated, it seems likely that the release of vasoactive substance, which is secreted by the ovaries under hCG stimulation, plays a key role in triggering this syndrome. Ovarian hyperstimulation syndrome occurs when ovulation-induction treatment results in the growth of multiple large follicles, massive extravascular protein-rich fluid shifts and secondary intravascular volume depletion.

The underlying mechanism responsible for the clinical manifestations of OHSS appears to be an increase in capillary permeability of the ovarian vessels and other mesothelial surfaces. It is the third-space fluid sequestration and the associated systemic vascular effects that contribute most to the morbidity and mortality associated with OHSS. The anatomical changes of the enlargement of the ovaries and the increased capillary permeability, which lead to acute fluid shift, may explain the different clinical features observed in this syndrome (Figure 1). Rapid body fluid shift in cases of ovarian hyperstimulation may lead to hypovolemia and hemoconcentration, as evidenced by increased hematocrit values and serum osmolarity. When not corrected immediately, hypovolemia may lead to decreased renal perfusion, subsequently stimulating the proximal renal tubules to resorb salt and water, resulting in clinical manifestations of oliguria, electrolyte imbalance and azotemia (Figure 2). The loss of fluid and protein into the peritoneal cavity and occasionally into the pleural cavity accounts for the hypovolemia and hemoconcentration that occurs. This in turn results in low blood pressure and decreased central venous pressure.

The dynamic fluid changes due to the vascular leak may lead to ascites, ARDS and to hemoconcentration and thromboembolic phenomena. The enlarged ovaries, composed of follicular and luteal cysts, may cause intraperitoneal bleeding or torsion, which require immediate surgical intervention.

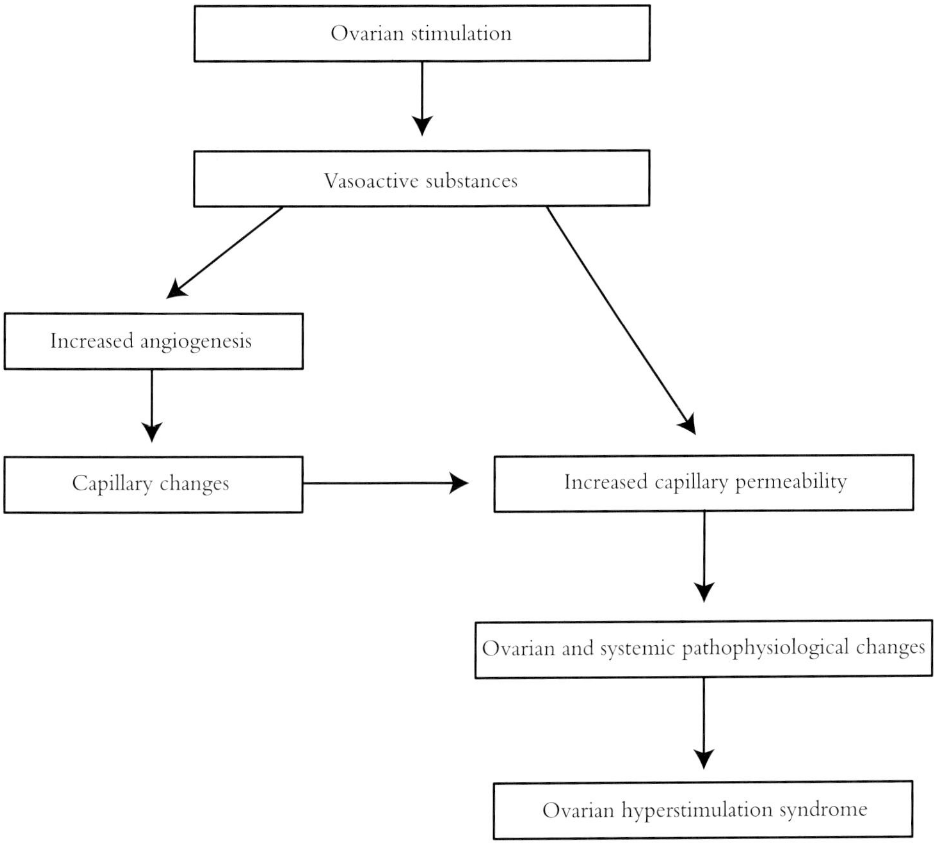

Figure 1 Pathophysiological changes in severe ovarian hyperstimulation syndrome

It is well established that removing the ascitic fluid by paracentesis dramatically improves the clinical condition of patients with severe OHSS; it results in improved renal and circulatory functions. This suggests that, in addition to biochemical factors, mechanical factors causing increasing intra-abdominal pressure, such as ascites and ovarian enlargement *per se*, could play an important role in the pathogenesis of OHSS[4,5].

Recently we observed clinical features additional to the ones published previously by us[1,2]. The objective of this study[6] was to define the incidence of febrile morbidity and its causes in severe and critical OHSS. For this purpose, we reviewed the medical records of all OHSS patients hospitalized in 16 out of 19 tertiary medical centers in Israel between January 1987 and December 1996. Febrile morbidity was defined as at least one episode of temperature rise above 38 °C lasting 24 h or longer.

A total of 2902 patients (3305 hospitalizations) with OHSS were identified, of whom 196 had severe, and 13 critical, OHSS. Among the 209 patients investigated, the

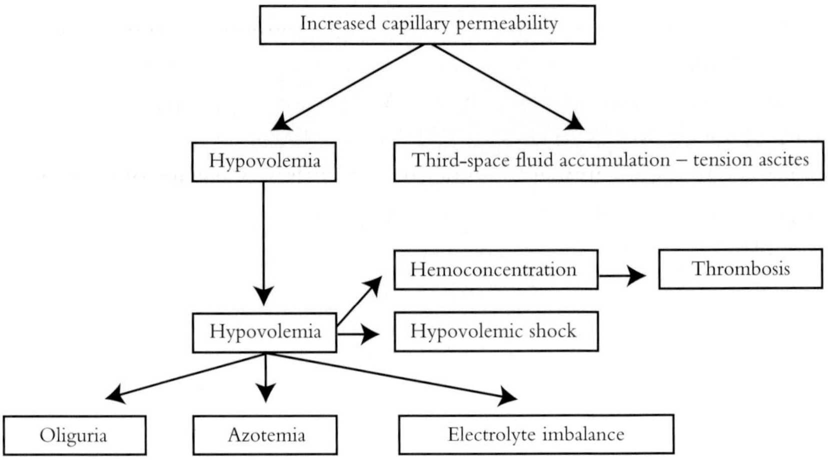

Figure 2 Basic changes leading to ovarian hyperstimulation syndrome

incidence of febrile morbidity was 82.3%, of which 20.5% was attributed to urinary tract infection, 3.8% to pneumonia, 3.3% to upper respiratory tract infection, 2.0% to intravenous-line phlebitis, 1.0% to cellulitis at an abdominal puncture site, 1.0% to postoperative wound infections and 0.5% to gluteal abscess at the site of progesterone injection. Non-typical organisms were frequently isolated, such as *Pseudomonas*, *Proteus*, *Klebsiella* and *Enterobacter* species. No infectious etiology was found in 105 patients (50.2%). Hypoglobulinemia was recorded in most patients, while ascitic and pleural fluids aspirated from these patients contained high globulin concentrations. We concluded that infection-related febrile morbidity in severe and critical OHSS is high, and may be attributed to some degree of immunodeficiency associated with loss of plasma globulins into the third space. However, non-infection-related febrile morbidity is higher and may be attributed to endogenous pyrogenic mechanisms.

An investigation was undertaken to assess immunoglobulin (Ig) concentrations in the plasma and ascitic fluid of patients with severe OHSS. Ten patients with severe OHSS after ovulation induction for *in vitro* fertilization (IVF) and ten controls who had undergone similar ovulation induction and did not develop OHSS were studied. Three blood samples were obtained from each OHSS patient: one at the time of hospitalization for severe OHSS, one when significant clinical improvement was evident and one at the first follow-up visit after discharge from the hospital. Blood samples were drawn from control patients 6–8 days after embryo transfer. Ascitic fluid was obtained from all patients with OHSS by therapeutic paracentesis. Immunoglobulin concentrations were assessed by radial immunodiffusion.

Significantly lower levels of γ globulins, specifically IgG and IgA, were detected in the plasma of patients with severe OHSS, whereas α- and β-globulin levels, as well as IgM levels, were not significantly different from those in controls. Both IgG and IgA levels increased as patients clinically improved. Ascitic fluid contained high IgG, moderate IgA and negligible IgM levels. The conclusion of our study was that severe OHSS is characterized by hypogammaglobulinemia, attributed to leakage of medium-molecular-weight immunoglobulins, such as IgG and IgA, into the peritoneal cavity[7].

Pathophysiology

Although the pathophysiology of this syndrome has not been completely elucidated, it seems likely that the increased capillary permeability triggered by the release of vasoactive substance, which is secreted by the ovaries under hCG stimulation, plays a key role in this syndrome. Several factors, such as histamine, serotonin, prostaglandin, prolactin and a variety of other substances, have been implicated in this process in the past. At present, factors belonging to the renin–angiotensin system, cytokines (including the interleukins), tumor necrosis factor-α (TNF-α), endothelin-1 and vascular endothelial growth factor are thought to be involved in triggering increased vascular permeability after ovulation-induction treatment.

Factors previously implicated in the pathogenesis of OHSS

Histamine and OHSS

It was found in rabbits that OHSS could be blocked by the administration of antihistamine preparations. In animals treated with antihistamine, a more rapid regression of the hyperstimulated ovaries was observed than in a control group. Although these animal studies had promising results, later studies demonstrated no difference in histamine levels between rabbits in which OHSS was induced and controls[8].

Estrogen and OHSS

Abnormally high levels of various steroids, estrogens in particular, are found in ascitic fluid and serum in cases of OHSS following hMG–hCG ovulation induction. Thus, it is not surprising that estrogens have been implicated as a possible triggering factor that eventually increases capillary permeability. It has been confirmed that this syndrome only develops after ovulation and corpus luteum formation. Experimental evidence in the rat and in the rabbit has shown that excessive estrogens may cause increased capillary permeability of the uterus and ovarian vessels.

On the other hand, it is known that high doses of estrogens do not, by themselves, produce clinical hyperstimulation. Moreover, Meirow and colleagues[9] described a case of OHSS in a patient with late-onset congenital adrenal hyperplasia after ovulation-induction treatment without any elevation of estrogen levels. Another indication estrogen is an 'innocent bystander' in OHSS is that, in experimental animals, the syndrome is not prevented by extraperitonealization of the ovaries[5]. Therefore, it is assumed that the increased capillary permeability found in cases of OHSS is due to some excess of immediate metabolites secreted by the ovary after hMG–hCG stimulation, rather than high estrogen levels *per se*.

Prostaglandins and OHSS

Experiments using animal models have been undertaken to determine whether prostaglandins are 'active substances' playing a role in the development of this syndrome. It was demonstrated in early experiments using an animal model that indomethacin, a blocker of prostaglandin synthesis, can prevent the fluid shift associated with the ascites, pleural effusion and hypovolemia seen in this syndrome[5]. Excessive estrogen produced by the large number of developing follicles may also stimulate increased production of prostaglandins, which in turn could be responsible for the increased capillary permeability observed in OHSS. In the clinical setting, indomethacin has been used as a therapeutic measure in cases of severe OHSS with variable results.

Human chorionic gonadotropin and OHSS

It is well known that the development of severe OHSS is dependent on either the exogenous administration of hCG or else endogenous pregnancy-derived hCG stimulation.

Human chorionic gonadotropin is administered during ovarian stimulation for both triggering ovulation and for luteal support. It is well known that hCG administration is critical for the development of OHSS. OHSS will not occur following administration of hMG alone, except in sporadic cases.

Human chorionic gonadotropin is also used for luteal-phase supplementation during gonadotropin releasing hormone agonist-controlled ovarian-hyperstimulated cycles. It was found that hCG administration could significantly increase the risk of OHSS. Thus, it was suggested that, whenever during controlled ovarian hyperstimulation estradiol levels are over 2500 pg/ml and the number of follicles exceeds ten, luteal support with hCG should be excluded.

Renin–angiotensin system and OHSS

Increased vascularity, as well as increased capillary permeability at the time of ovulation, is an important part of the angiogenic response in the follicle. The angiogenic properties of human follicular fluid, combined with high prorenin, high plasma renin-like activity, angiotensin II-like immunoreactivity and angiotensin converting enzyme in human follicular fluid, raised the idea of the possible involvement of the renin–angiotensin system in the pathogenesis of OHSS through new vessel formation and increased capillary permeability[10]. The involvement of a locally activated renin–angiotensin–aldosterone cascade has been implicated as a possible cause of the severe form of the syndrome through neovascularization and increased capillary permeability rate[11] (Figure 3).

We studied[10] plasma renin activity and aldosterone in patients with ovarian hyperstimulation and showed that the pattern of plasma renin activity in hMG-hyperstimulated cycles was characterized by a mid-luteal peak, which declined to normal in the late luteal phase in non-conceptual cycles, whereas a sustained elevation of plasma renin activity occurred in conceptual cycles. A direct correlation between the magnitude of plasma renin activity and the severity of OHSS was established. A significant correlation was demonstrated between plasma renin activity in the serum and either progesterone or estradiol levels. Elevated levels of plasma aldosterone were observed in cycles with OHSS and especially in conceptual cycles with OHSS.

Our study therefore showed that the increased capillary permeability present in OHSS was due to the involvement of the renin–angiotensin system and the synthesis of prostaglandins in the ovaries.

Interleukins in OHSS[12]

Recent work on ovarian physiology has suggested an interaction between the immune system and the ovaries. These findings may shed new light on understanding the pathophysiology of OHSS (Figure 4). Cytokines, polypeptide products of immune cells that have profound effects upon non-immune tissues, have been shown to play a role in the mediation of ovulation.

Interleukin I (IL-1)

IL-1, a polypeptide cytokine predominantly produced and secreted by activated macrophages, has been shown to possess a wide range of biological functions, as well as to play a role as an immune mediator. It plays an important role in the pathogenesis of

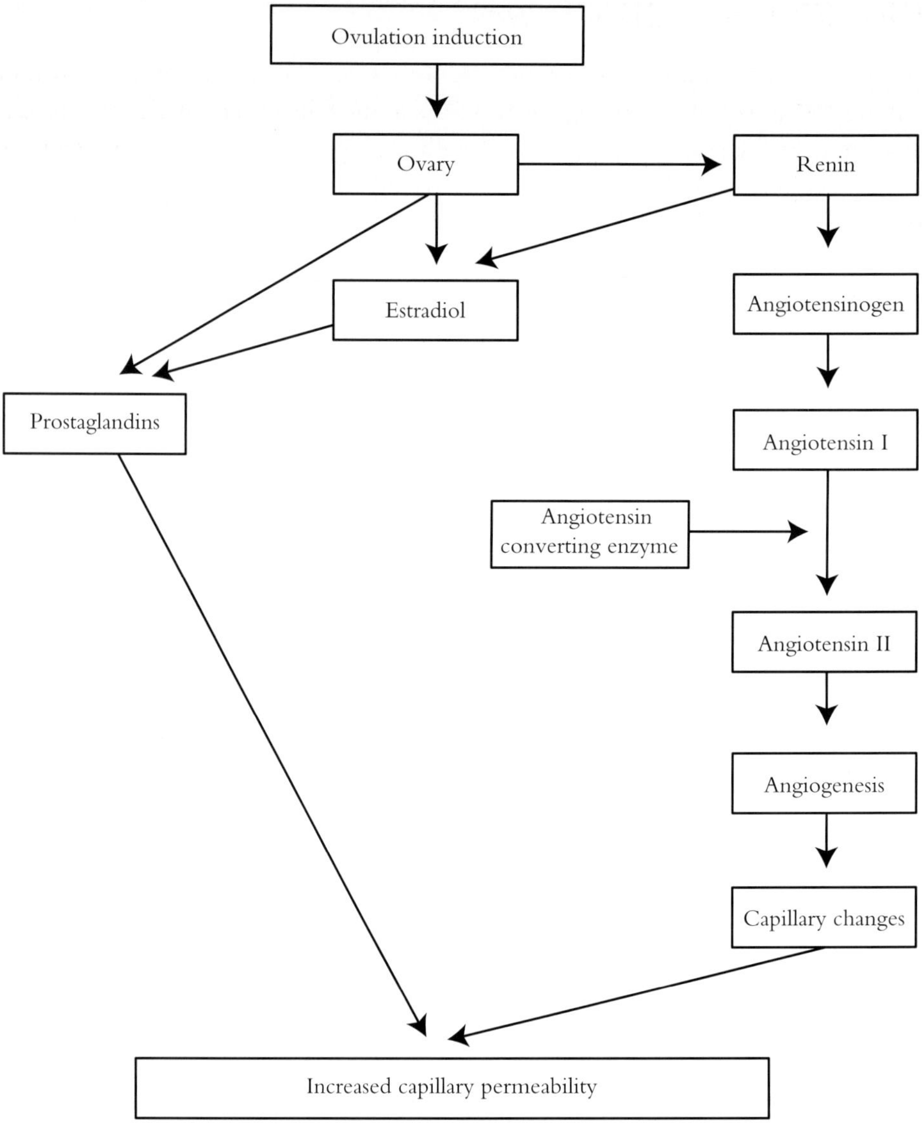

Figure 3 Suggested role of the angiotensin–renin system and prostaglandins in the pathogenesis of ovarian hyperstimulation syndrome

many diseases and mediates a broad spectrum of systemic changes involved in the host response to infection, inflammation, immunological challenge and injury. These facts, combined with evidence that IL-1 is implicated in ovulation, raised the possibility that IL-1 may be involved in OHSS as well. A significant decrease in IL-1 was observed with concurrent clinical resolution in patients with severe OHSS[5]. Hypothetically, IL-1 released to the systemic circulation during severe OHSS may cause capillary

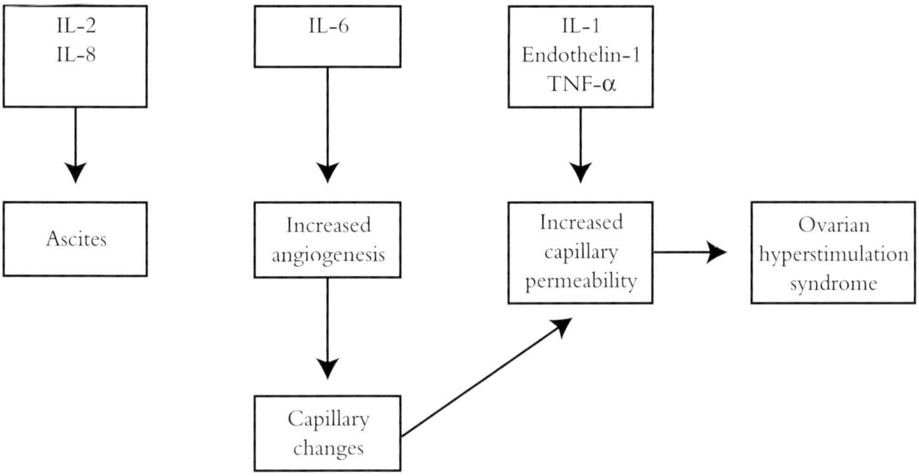

Figure 4 Suggested role of interleukins in ovarian hyperstimulation syndrome. IL, interleukin; TNF-α, tumor necrosis factor-α

hyperpermeability, hemoconcentration (as manifested by an elevated hematocrit) and possibly other acute-phase responses.

Interleukin 6 (IL-6)

Various types of lymphoid and non-lymphoid cells produce IL-6, including T cells, B cells, mesangium cells and several tumor cells. Elevated concentrations of IL-6 have been reported in some patients with septic shock, and elevated IL-6 levels have been correlated with hypotension, shock and mortality. Revel and colleagues[13] found a high IL-6 activity in the plasma and ascitic fluid of patients with OHSS. Recently, our group has also found high cytokine levels in the ascitic fluid and plasma of patients with OHSS[14]. Increased capillary permeability and neovascularization play a central role in the pathogenesis of OHSS. IL-6, along with IL-1 and TNF-α, mediate systemic reactions characterized by leukocytosis and increased vascular permeability, and increased levels of acute-phase proteins synthesized by the liver are characteristic of OHSS as well. The mechanism by which IL-6 might mediate the pathogenesis of this syndrome is not completely clear, although it might be involved in neovascularization and ascites formation.

TNF-α

TNF-α has an acute, concentration-dependent vasodilatory effect on vascular smooth muscle. A significantly increased TNF-α activity has been found in severe OHSS, followed by a fast decrease accompanying clinical resolution. These kinetics of plasma TNF-α suggest a possible role for TNF-α in the pathophysiology of OHSS.

Endothelin-1

Endothelin-1, an endothelial-derived peptide, is a potent vasoconstrictor that increases capillary permeability in several tissues. High levels of endothelin-1 were found in follicular fluid from patients undergoing ovulation induction. The Endothelin-1 concentration was found to be 100–300-fold higher in the follicular fluid than in the plasma. Moreover, a positive correlation between the concentrations of endothelin-1 and follicle stimulating hormone in the follicular fluid was found, suggesting that endothelin-1 may play a role in ovarian function as well as in OHSS.

Vascular endothelial growth factor

Vascular endothelial growth factor (VEGF) is a potent vasoactive protein with a remarkable permeability-enhancing capacity that is approximately 1000 times that of histamine. Follicular fluid VEGF concentration was found to be 100-fold greater than that in the serum or peritoneal fluid 36 h after hCG administration. Evidence for the key role of VEGF in the pathogenesis of OHSS was reported by our group[15] (Figure 5). To assess the potential involvement of VEGF in the hyperpermeability characterizing OHSS, a controlled clinical study that followed the kinetics of VEGF in the plasma of patients with severe OHSS from the time of admission to the hospital until clinical resolution was carried out. Seven women hospitalized in a tertiary medical center who had severe OHSS after ovulation induction for IVF, and seven controls who had received a similar ovulation-induction regimen and did not develop OHSS, were studied. Three blood samples were obtained from each OHSS patient: the first upon hospitalization for severe OHSS, the second when significant clinical improvement was evident and the third on the first follow-up visit after the patient's discharge. Ascitic fluid was obtained from all OHSS patients by therapeutic paracentesis during the active phase of the syndrome. Blood samples were drawn from the control patients 4–6 days after embryo transfer. VEGF levels, hematocrit, estradiol levels and white blood cell count were determined for all samples. VEGF levels were established by enzyme-linked immunosorbent assay and estradiol levels were determined by radioimmunoassay. Compared to the controls, high levels of VEGF were detected in the plasma of all patients admitted for severe OHSS. Levels dropped significantly with clinical improvement, reaching minimum values after complete resolution. A statistically significant correlation was found between plasma VEGF levels and certain biological characteristics of OHSS and capillary leakage, such as leukocytosis and increased hematocrit. Ascitic fluid obtained from the study patients also contained high levels of VEGF.

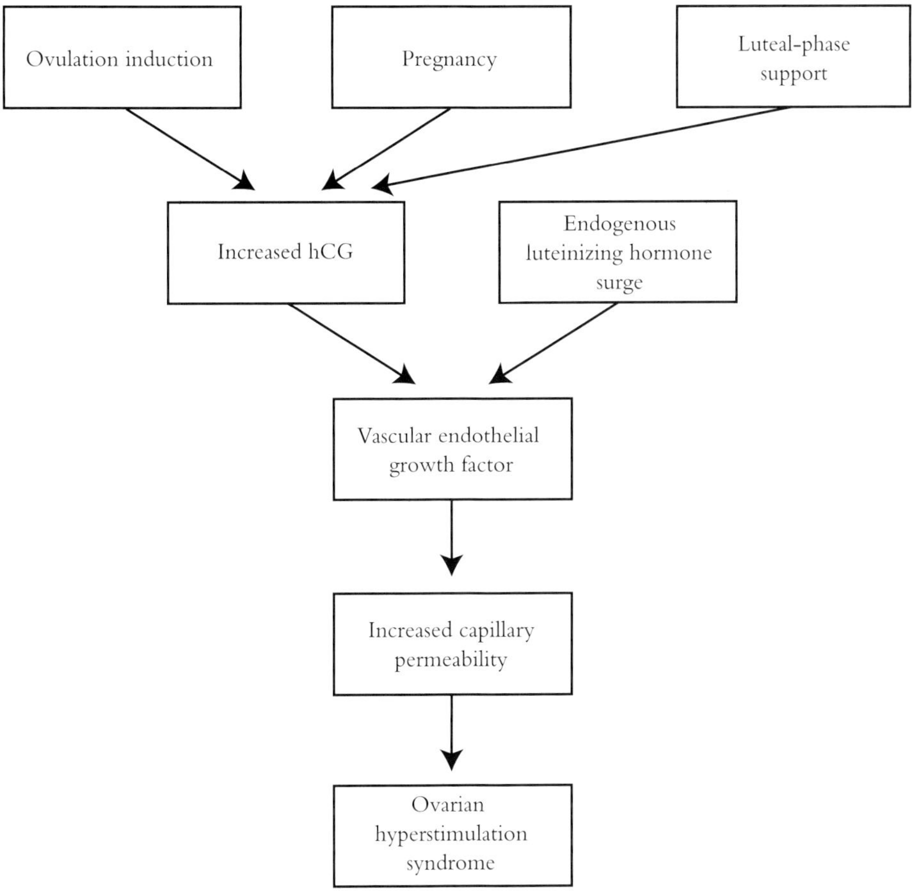

Figure 5 Suggested role of vascular endothelial growth factor in ovarian hyperstimulation syndrome. hCG, human chorionic gonadotropin

These findings suggest that VEGF is involved in the pathogenesis of capillary leakage in OHSS.

RISK OF MALIGNANCY

Risk of epithelial ovarian cancer

To determine whether women with epithelial ovarian cancer are more likely to have been exposed to fertility drugs (in particular hMG) than healthy population controls, a nationwide case–control study was carried out[16]. A total of 200 women, 36–64 years of age, with a histologically confirmed diagnosis of primary invasive or borderline epithelial ovarian cancer that was first diagnosed and reported to the Israel Cancer Registry between 1 January 1990 and 1 September 1993 were enrolled. There were 164 (82%)

invasive and 36 (18%) borderline epithelial ovarian tumors among the 200 cases. The controls were 408 women from the same telephone dialling areas selected by random-digit dialling. Cases and controls were interviewed using a standard questionnaire. A multivariate logistic model was used to assess the association of fertility drug use and ovarian cancer, controlling for variables found to be statistically associated with this outcome on univariate analysis. Twenty-four women with epithelial ovarian cancer (12%) and 29 healthy controls (7.1%) reported that they had used any fertility drug (adjusted odds ratio (OR) 1.31, 95% confidence interval (CI) 0.63–2.74). Among cases and controls, respectively, 22 and 24 reported that they had used hMG alone or in combination with clomiphene citrate (adjusted OR 1.42, 95% CI 0.65–3.12), and 11 and six reported that they had used hMG alone (adjusted OR 3.19, 95% CI 0.86–11.82). The risk was particularly increased in the subgroup of women with borderline ovarian tumors who had used hMG (adjusted OR 9.38, 95% CI 1.66–52.08). We concluded that the use of ovulation-induction agents, in particular hMG, may increase the risk of epithelial ovarian tumors.

Breast cancer

The results of both epidemiological and experimental studies suggest that endogenous (and apparently exogenous) sex hormones and other reproductive variables have an important role in the development of human breast neoplasms. Nevertheless, no controlled study has ever addressed the possible effects of ovarian stimulation on the incidence and course of human breast cancer. Over the past decade, the number of women undergoing follicular stimulation, especially during assisted reproductive technology procedures, has grown rapidly. A study has been published in which 16 young women who were treated by ovulation induction were subsequently diagnosed with breast cancer. These women were identified out of 950 cases of infertile women who underwent ovulation induction at our fertility clinic over a 10-year period. The possible association between ovarian stimulation and the promotion of breast cancer has been discussed and the need for a controlled study was emphasized[17].

OBSTETRIC COMPLICATIONS

Spontaneous abortion rate

Pregnancies achieved by assisted reproduction are considered to carry increased risk for spontaneous abortion, as well as ectopic and heterotopic pregnancies. In order to examine the validity of this hypothesis, we compared the outcomes of spontaneous pregnancies and assisted reproduction pregnancies using the published reports in the world literature over the past decade[18]. We also studied the outcomes of 153 000 IVF pregnancies. The reported loss rates (abortions and ectopic pregnancies) in spontaneous pregnancies compared to pregnancies achieved by assisted reproduction were 19% and 30%, respectively. The differences in loss rates between spontaneous and assisted reproduction pregnancies are not completely understood and may originate from predisposing factors, such as tubal disease, uterine disorders, corpus luteum dysfunction and endometriosis, being more frequent in patients suffering from infertility. Increasing maternal age correlates with a higher risk of fetal chromosomal anomalies, which results in an increased rate of abortions.

Heterotopic pregnancy

Heterotopic pregnancy, an extremely rare event in the past, has become a common complication of assisted reproduction techniques. This serious sequel to *in vitro* fertilization–embryo transfer or gamete intra-Fallopian transfer is probably the result of ovarian hyperstimulation and the transfer of several embryos into the uterus or tubes of a preselected population suffering from mechanical infertility. The techniques and medium used for embryo transfer may also be involved. Delayed diagnosis resulting in rupture, hemorrhage and emergency intervention, with its serious consequences, is being reported in nearly half of the cases. The prognosis for a viable intrauterine pregnancy, however, is good and these combined pregnancies have produced a living child in about 70% of cases[19]. A high index of suspicion, ultrasound examinations and early intervention are mandatory to salvage the viable intrauterine pregnancy and avoid maternal mortality.

Pregnancy outcome in OHSS[14]

To assess the outcome of pregnancies conceived with the use of IVF that are complicated by severe OHSS, a retrospective[14] nationwide multicenter study was carried out in 16 of the 19 tertiary-care medical centers in Israel. All patients undergoing IVF who were hospitalized for severe OHSS between January 1987 and December 1996 were studied. Pregnancy rate and rates of multiple gestation, miscarriage, ectopic pregnancy, obstetric complications and intervention were evaluated. A total of 163 patients who had severe OHSS after IVF treatment were identified, of whom 142 (87.1%) had undergone embryo transfer. The clinical pregnancy rate was 73.2%; 42.3% of pregnancies were singletons, 33.6% were twins, 17.3% were triplets and 6.7% were quadruplets. The miscarriage rate was 29.8%, whereas the incidence of ectopic pregnancy was 1.9%. Forty-four per cent of all births were premature and 62.1% of all newborns had a low birth weight. The most common antenatal complications were pregnancy-induced hypertension (13.2%), gestational diabetes (5.9%) and placental abruption (4.4%). The rate of Cesarean section was 44.1%. Among patients who had severe OHSS after IVF treatment, the pregnancy rate and the rates of multiple gestation, miscarriage, prematurity, low birth weight, pregnancy-induced hypertension, gestational diabetes and placental abruption were significantly higher than those reported previously for pregnancies conceived with the use of assisted reproductive techniques.

REFERENCES

1. Schenker JG, Polishuk WZ. Ascites in cases of twin pregnancy. *J Obstet Gynaecol Br Commonw* 1967;74:451–2
2. Schenker JG, Weinstein D. Ovarian hyperstimulation syndrome: a current survey. *Fertil Steril* 1978;30:255–68
3. Schenker JG. Prevention and treatment of ovarian hyperstimulation. *Hum Reprod* 1993;8:653–9
4. Schenker JG, Polishuk WZ. The role of prostaglandins in ovarian hyperstimulation syndrome. *Eur J Obstet Gynecol Reprod Biol* 1976;6:47–52
5. Polishuk WZ, Schenker JG. Ovarian overstimulation syndrome. *Fertil Steril* 1969;20:433–50
6. Abramov Y, Elchalal U, Schenker JG. Febrile morbidity in severe and critical ovarian hyperstimulation syndrome: a multicentre study. *Hum Reprod* 1998;13:3128–31
7. Abramov Y, Naparstek Y, Elchalal U, Lewin A, Schechter E, Schenker JG. Plasma immunoglobulins in patients with severe ovarian hyperstimulation syndrome. *Fertil Steril* 1999;71:102–5
8. Knox GE. Antihistamine blockade of the ovarian hyperstimulation syndrome. *Am J Obstet Gynecol* 1974;118:992–4
9. Meirow D, Schenker JG, Rosler A. Ovarian hyperstimulation syndrome with low estradiol in non classic 17alpha-hydroxylase, 17,20-lyase deficiency: what is the role of estrogens? *Hum Reprod* 1996;11:2119–21
10. Navot D, Margalioth EJ, Laufer N, *et al.* Direct correlation between plasma renin activity and severity of ovarian hyperstimulation syndrome. *Fertil Steril* 1987;48:57–61
11. Mordel N, Schenker JG. Gonadotropin releasing hormone agonist and ovarian hyperstimulation syndrome in assisted reproduction. *Hum Reprod* 1993;8:2009–201
12. Abramov Y, Schenker JG, Lewin A, Friedler S, Nisman B, Barak V. Plasma inflammatory cytokines correlate to the ovarian hyperstimulation syndrome. *Hum Reprod* 1996;11: 1381–6
13. Revel A, Barak Y, Lavy Y, *et al.* Characterization of intraperitoneal cytokines and nitrites in women with severe ovarian hyperstimulation syndrome. *Fertil Steril* 1996;66:66–71
14. Abramov Y, Elchalal U, Schenker JG. Obstetric outcome of *in vitro* fertilized pregnancies complicated by severe ovarian hyperstimulation syndrome: a multicenter study. *Fertil Steril* 1998;70:1070–6
15. Abramov Y, Barak V, Nisman B, Schenker JG. Vascular endothelial growth factor plasma levels correlate to the clinical picture in severe ovarian hyperstimulation syndrome. *Fertil Steril* 1997;67:261–5

16. Shushan A, Paltiel O, Iscovich J, Elchalal U, Peretz T, Schenker JG. Human menopausal gonadotropin and the risk of epithelial ovarian cancer. *Fertil Steril* 1996;6:13–18
17. Brzezinski A, Peretz T, Mor-Yosef S, Schenker JG. Ovarian stimulation and breast cancer: is there a link? *Gynecol Oncol* 1994;52:292–5
18. Ezra Y, Schenker JG. Abortion rate in assisted reproduction – true increase? *Early Pregnancy* 1995;1:171–5
19. Rojansky N, Schenker JG. Heterotopic pregnancy and assisted reproduction – an update. *J Assist Reprod Genet* 1996;13:594–601

Menopause

7

Steroid hormones and the central nervous system

M. Neves-e-Castro

The central nervous system (CNS) and steroid hormones are two enormous and complex fields of modern physiology, with a very rapid and intensive accumulation of new data and novel concepts. The study of the hormonal modulation of CNS functions is an even more complicated endeavor. The precise extrapolation from neuroanatomy and neurobiochemistry into mental performance is a very difficult task in view of so many external confounding factors.

In vitro experiments and *in vivo* studies in animals, as well as the visualization of mental performance in humans with the help of new dynamic imaging techniques, are opening new horizons in the understanding of the effects of hormone deprivation and replacement on human psychological functioning. The published observations are so abundant that it is not easy accurately to review all of them. Nevertheless, there are some well-established findings:

(1) The brain has well-identified anatomical structures that are related to defined motor, sensitive and psychological functions. This was established through experimentally induced stereotaxic lesions in animals or by the localization of traumatic or tumoral lesions in the human brain.

(2) *In vitro* studies with cell cultures from different cerebral nuclei have identified several molecules that were shown to act as neurotransmitters within the neuronal network.

(3) Histochemical studies have characterized the predominant localization of these neurotransmitters in certain nuclei and zones of the brain.

(4) The pharmacological modulation of such neurotransmitters (release, uptake, etc.) causes changes in psychological functions (mood, memory, cognition, etc.).

(5) Sex steroid hormones interfere with brain neurotransmitters. They act by genomic and non-genomic mechanisms. In doing so, they affect mental performance.

(6) Sex steroid hormones have nerve growth factor-like activity in neuronal cell cultures.

(7) Using positron emission tomography and dynamic magnetic resonance imaging, brain function has been visualized during tests of mental performance and has been shown to be affected by the administration of steroid hormones.

(8) Hormone replacement therapy (HRT) improves brain circulation, decreases lipoprotein oxidation and protects the brain from oxygen free radicals.

(9) HRT in postmenopausal women, or after castration, improves mood and mental performance with restoration to almost normal function.

(10) Postmenopausal women being treated with long-term HRT have some degree of protection from depression and dementia, and have better cognition, memory and sleep quality.

(11) Every practitioner experienced in the administration of HRT to postmenopausal women is well aware of the fact that, other than the relief of vasomotor symptoms, the first improvement noticed and reported by these women is in their mood, mental performance and quality of life.

Hundreds of studies could be quoted in support of each of the above statements. Instead, reference shall only be made to some of the more updated and comprehensive reviews as a source of important information.

For the clinician, what matters in a very pragmatic way is that the HRT he knows should be prescribed for the primary and secondary prevention of cardiovascular diseases and osteoporosis has another very important additional benefit at the CNS level, again for both symptom relief and primary/secondary prevention. In postmenopausal women, the overall benefit/risk assessment of HRT is well established. Be it for primary or secondary prevention, in addition to symptom relief, it is nowadays accepted as being a standard of good clinical practice.

The theoretical discussion of the validity of many epidemiological studies, as well as a number of clinical trials and *in vitro* studies, on the effects of steroid hormones on the CNS is no doubt very important. Nevertheless, the recommended doses for HRT will remain the same. The schemes of administration will not change. The reasons for using HRT may be increased, but certainly not decreased, no matter what the practitioner thinks about the effect of estrogens on the CNS.

In practical terms, what is already known today about this fascinating new field will certainly aid the practitioner in explaining to his clients another major reason why they should start and adhere to long-lasting HRT under usual medical supervision. HRT has definite positive effects on CNS function and on the prevention of disease, in both the short and the long term.

BIBLIOGRAPHY

Birge SJ, ed. The role of ovarian hormones in cognition and dementia. *Neurology* 1997; 48(Suppl 7)

Genazzani AR, Petraglia F, Purdy RH, eds. *The Brain: Source and Target for Sex Steroid Hormones*. Carnforth, UK: Parthenon Publishing, 1996

McEwen BS. Clinical review 108: the molecular and neuroanatomical basis for estrogen effects in the central nervous system. *J Clin Endocrinol Metab* 1999;84:1790–7

McEwen BS, Alves SE. Estrogen actions in the central nervous system. *Endocr Rev* 1999;20: 279–307

Wise PM, Smith MJ, Dubal DB, *et al.* Neuroendocrine influences and repercussions of the menopause. *Endocr Rev* 1999;20:243–8

Toran-Allerand CD, Singh M, Setalo G Jr. Novel mechanisms of estrogen action in the brain: new players in an old story. *Front Neuroendocrinol* 1999;20:97–121

Pike CJ. Estrogen modulates neuronal *Bcl-xL* expression and β-amyloid-induced apoptosis: relevance to Alzheimer's disease. *J Neurochem* 1999;72:1552–63

Bethea CL, Pecins-Thompson M, Schutzer WE, *et al.* Ovarian steroids and serotonin neural function. *Mol Neurobiol* 1998;18:87–123

Dubal DB, Kashon ML, Pettigrew LC, *et al.* Estradiol protects against ischemic injury. *J Cereb Blood Flow Metab* 1998;18:1253–8

Gibbs RB, Aggarwal P. Estrogen and basal forebrain cholinergic neurons: implications for brain aging and Alzheimer's disease-related cognitive decline. *Horm Behav* 1998;34:98–111

Kuiper GG, Shughrue PJ, Merchenthaler I, *et al.* The estrogen receptor beta subtype: a novel mediator of estrogen action in neuroendocrine systems. *Front Neuroendocrinol* 1998;19: 253–86

Fink G, Sumner BE, McQueen JK, *et al.* Sex steroid control of mood, mental state and memory. *Clin Exp Pharmacol Physiol* 1998;25:764–75

Yaffe K, Sawaya G, Lieberburg I, *et al.* Estrogen therapy in postmenopausal women: effects on cognitive function and dementia. *J Am Med Assoc* 1998;279:688–95

Brinton RD, Tran J, Proffitt P, *et al.* 17β-Estradiol enhances the outgrowth and survival of neocortical neurons in culture. *Neurochem Res* 1997;22:1339–51

Baulieu EE, Schumacher M. Neurosteroids, with special reference to the effect of progesterone on myelination in peripheral nerves. *Mult Scler* 1997;3:105–12

Berman KF, Schmidt PJ, Rubinow DR, *et al.* Modulation of cognition-specific cortical activity by gonadal steroids: a positron-emission tomography study in women. *Proc Natl Acad Sci USA* 1997;94:8836–41

Shaywitz SE, Shaywitz BA, Pugh KR, *et al.* Effect of estrogen on brain activation patterns in postmenopausal women during working memory tasks. *J Am Med Assoc* 1999;281: 1197–202

Inestrosa NC, Marzolo MP, Bonnefont AB. Cellular and molecular basis of estrogen's neuroprotection. Potential relevance for Alzheimer's disease. *Mol Neurobiol* 1998;17:73–86

Sherwin BB. Estrogen and cognitive functioning in women. *Proc Soc Exp Biol Med* 1998; 217:17–22

Sherwin BB. Cognitive assessment for postmenopausal women and general assessment of their mental health. *Psychopharmacol Bull* 1998;34:323–6

8

Primary and preventive osteoporosis care

M. Brincat, R. Galea and Y. Muscat Baron

INTRODUCTION

Collagen is the major protein component of most connective tissues of vertebrates. In mammals it constitutes approximately 25–35% of their total protein. It is present in virtually each and every animal tissue, providing an extracellular framework for all metazoan animals. It is a highly conserved, evolutionarily ancient family of molecules.

Collagens are a large family of proteins; this family is made up of at least 19 different members, which are found in human tissues. These are made up of about 30 distinct polypeptide chains. There are the same number of genes that encode procollagen polypeptides.

Collagen molecules are characterized by the formation of three left-handed polypeptide helical chains that are tightly coiled around each other in a rope-like fashion to form a right-handed supercoil. The collagen helix is more extended than an α-helix, since it has 3.0 amino-acid residues per turn, with a pitch of 0.94 nm, giving a rise of 0.31 nm per residue. All collagens contain greater or lesser stretches of this triple helix.

Type I collagen, which constitutes 90% of the total collagen in the body, is the most important[1]. It is predominant in skin and bone. In addition to type I collagen, skin also contains some of the very similar type III collagen.

Bone and skin are the two organs that together contain 80% of all the connective tissues found in the human body. Both show a deterioration with estrogen deficiency. This deterioration can be prevented, and even reversed, with appropriate and adequate estrogen replacement[2–5].

BONE

Bone is a dynamic structure. It is made up of both organic and inorganic material. In the past, postmenopausal studies have mainly concentrated on the inorganic component, ignoring the organic one. The main organic matter is protein, of which there are two main types: the collagens and the non-collagen proteins.

The collagens are mainly type I collagen, with type V making up a minor component. The non-collagen proteins include plasma proteins, proteoglycans, osteocalcin, osteonectin and bone sialoprotein. Collagens make up the greatest proportion, as they constitute approximately 35% of the dry defatted bone mass. The organic matrix of bone acts rather like internal girders and confers on bone its tensile strength. It has been suggested that it is a decline in this organic matrix that is the primary pathological event leading to osteoporosis[6,7].

Since bone is a living structure, it is being remodelled throughout our entire life. This remodelling is brought about at a cellular level by bone resorbing cells, the osteoclasts, and bone forming cells, the osteoblasts. The osteoclasts and osteoblasts remove and replace small quantities of bone at certain points throughout the skeleton. Bone mass at any point in life represents the balance attained between the peak bone mass laid down by the fourth decade of life and the amount of bone lost with aging. This loss of bone is an age-related loss in both sexes, but in women there is an acceleration in the rate of bone loss following the menopause. It has been shown[8] that, by the age of 70 years, women lose up to 50% of their bone mass, while a man would be expected to lose only 25% by the age of 90.

In order to investigate the relationship between age, bone mass and skin thickness, our group carried out a study on postmenopausal women. This consisted of a biophysical study that looked at differences in various bone density patterns on skin thickness measurements. Bone was measured using a dual energy X-ray absorptiometer (between lumbar vertebrae 2 and 4, at the femur neck and at Ward's triangle), while skin thickness was measured using high-frequency (22 MHz) ultrasound. The latter correlates with the collagen content in the skin. These measurements were carried out on a group of untreated postmenopausal women and a group of untreated postmenopausal women who had sustained an osteoporotic fracture. The results showed that the skin thickness and bone density parameters were much lower in women who had sustained osteoporotic fractures than in the controls (Figure 1).

Women with fractures had mean bone mass values that were 20% below the mean values of controls. Skin thickness varied within a narrower range (mean difference 4%), but significant differences between controls and women who had sustained an osteoporotic fracture were also consistently noted. When the skin thickness measurements were combined with bone density parameters, the accuracy of trying to predict an osteoporotic fracture was increased, as shown in Figure 2[9].

Bone has been shown to be an estradiol-responsive tissue and, in women, a hypoestrogenemic state leads to increased bone loss, especially in the first few years of estrogen deprivation. This is probably caused by an increase in the number and activity of osteoclasts. Estrogen has, in fact, been shown to inhibit, at a cellular level, the differentiation of osteoclasts. This results in a decrease in the number and activity of osteoclasts. The mechanism of action is probably mediated via some cytokines, most probably interleukin (IL)-1 and IL-6. It is known that estrogen regulates the expression of IL-6 in the bone marrow cells. The action modality is not known. On the other hand, the effect of estrogen on osteoblasts (the bone-forming cells) may either be a direct effect or it may rely on an alteration of the coupling phenomenon of bone formation and bone resorption[10].

Estrogen replacement affects osteoporosis in two ways: it can either prevent it or else it can treat the condition once it has occurred. It has been postulated that estrogen replacement therapy leads to an increase in bone mass by increasing the collagen levels in bone. Indeed, the observation that women on estrogen replacement therapy have a higher dermal skin collagen content than those who are not on estrogen replacement therapy has led to the idea that a similar increase in bone collagen content in women on estrogen replacement therapy occurs. It is possibly this increase in collagen content that leads to an increase in bone strength and thus a diminution of osteoporotic fractures. When estrogens are started in the menopausal period and continued into late life, the best results concerning bone density are obtained. However, if estrogen therapy is initiated later on in life, the benefits obtained are also good[11].

In order to investigate the collagen changes occurring with estrogen therapy, our group undertook another study[12]. This study was a biophysical/biochemical study comparing a group of untreated postmenopausal women and a group of women who were on estrogen replacement therapy. Apart from undergoing the same bone density and skin thickness measurements as in the previous study (mentioned above), the women in this study also had estimations of collagen marker excretion carried out.

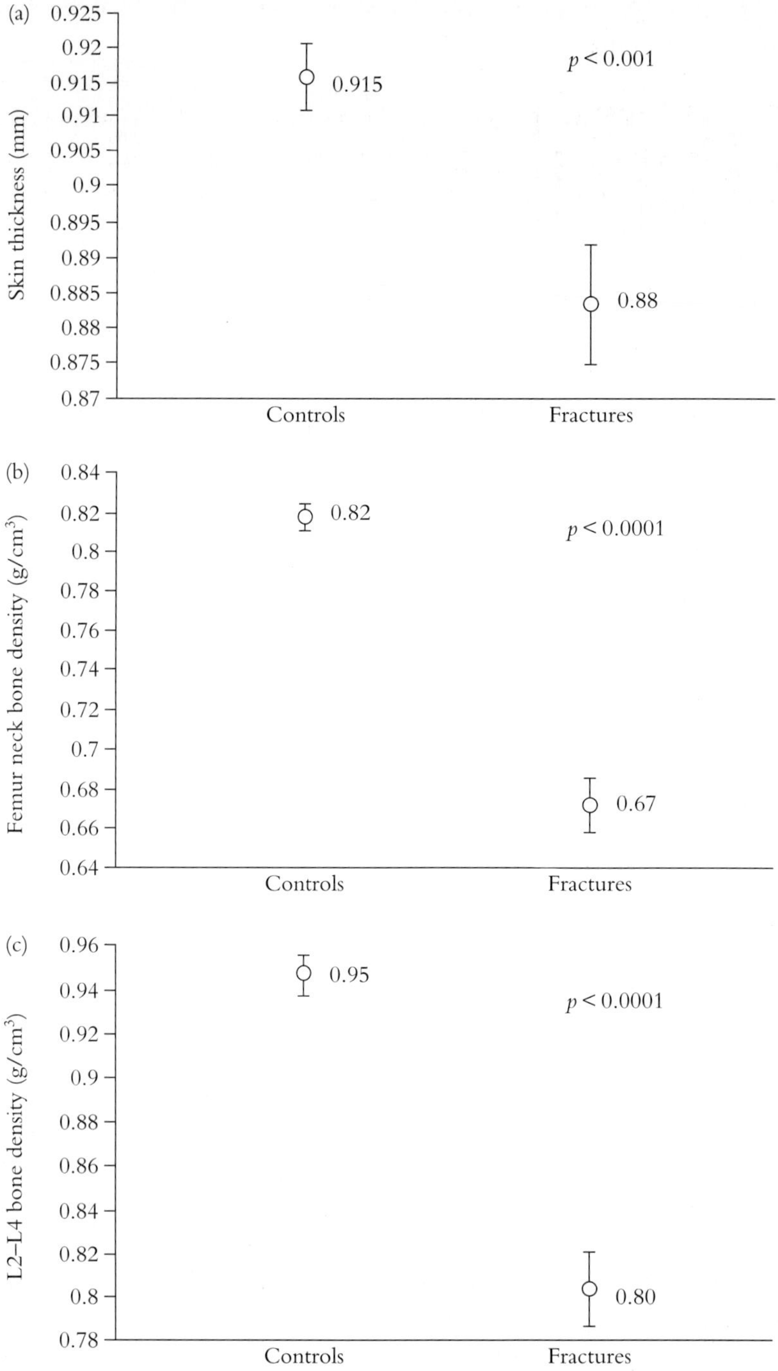

Figure 1 Plots (mean ± SE) of (a) skin thickness, (b) femur neck bone density and (c) L2–L4 bone density in patients with osteoporotic fractures (n = 411) and controls (n = 119)

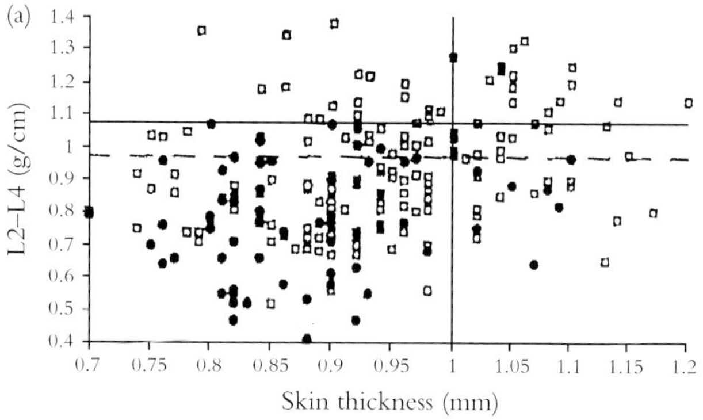

	Sensitivity	*Accuracy*
Skin thickness	91.8%	38.7%
L2–L4	100%	39.6%
Box L2–L4	91.8%	50.1%

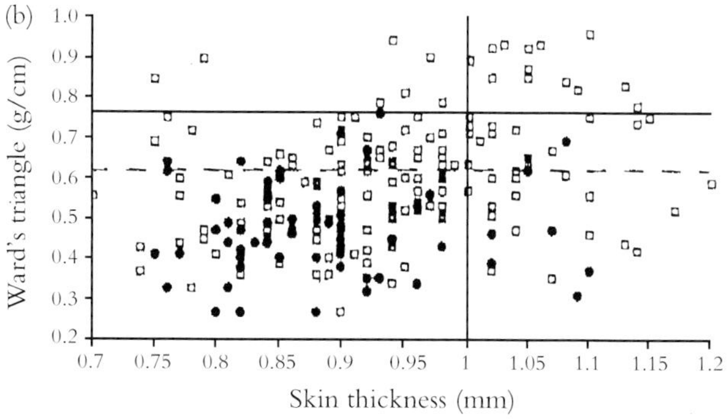

	Sensitivity	*Accuracy*
Skin thickness	91.7%	39.2%
Ward's triangle	100%	50.9%
Box Ward's triangle	91.7%	59.1%

Figure 2 Scattergrams for (a) L2–L4 versus skin thickness and (b) Ward's triangle versus skin thickness, in patients with osteoporotic fractures (●; n = 129) and controls (□; n = 411)

In this study we looked at the excretion of procollagen I C-terminal peptides (PCICP), a marker for bone formation, and pyridinium cross-links, a marker for bone resorption. When the untreated postmenopausal controls were compared with the women who had been on hormone replacement therapy, the latter showed a drastic decrease in osteoclastic activity (excretion of pyridinium cross-links). The mean decrease was in the order of 27.2%. There was also a decrease in bone formation, the osteoblastic activity (serum procollagen I C-terminal peptide) being decreased by a mean of 11.3%. All these differences ($p < 0.001$) indicated that bone remodelling had altered in the patients on estrogen replacement therapy. The women in this study were who were taking hormone replacement therapy had only been on this treatment for a short time (mean 6 months). This may imply that changes occur rapidly. It is interesting to note that, according to the above calculations based on bone collagen markers, a mean positive change of 15.9% occurred in bone remodelling in the women on estrogen replacement therapy. This value is of the same order as the mean percentage change in bone mass of the same women, measured using a biophysical method. This showed a mean positive change of 16.1% in the lumbar vertebra (L)2–L4 region[12] (Figure 3).

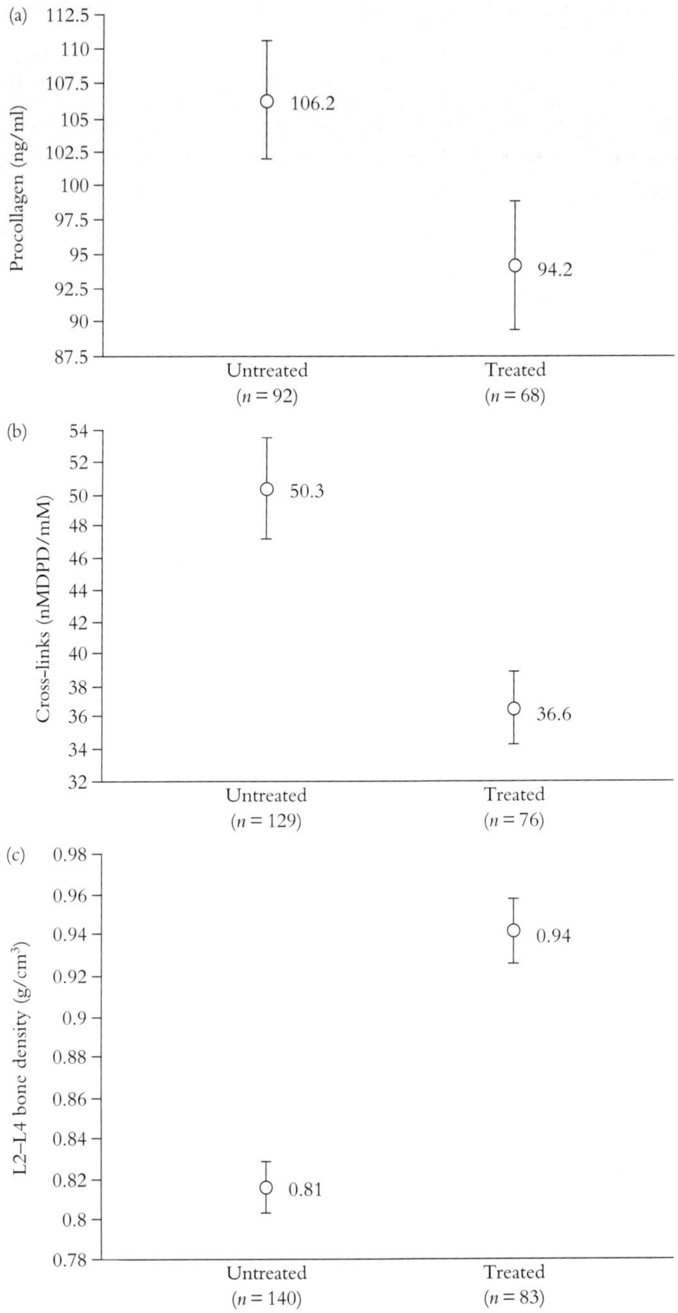

Figure 3 Plots (mean ± SE) of (a) procollagen, (b) cross-links and (c) L2–L4 bone density in untreated patients and in patients on hormone replacement therapy. There was an 11.3% change ($p < 0.05$) in bone formation (a), a 27.2% change ($p < 0.005$) in bone resorption (b) and a 16.1% change ($p < 0.001$) in bone density in the L2–L4 region (c) in the treated compared to the untreated patients

This could indicate that these markers are, indeed, sensitive and can be used in monitoring postmenopausal bone loss, as well as accurately titrating the response to treatment, both when such treatment is prophylactic and also when it is used therapeutically in the management of established osteoporosis. The excretion of pyridinium collagen cross-links in first-void morning urine samples shows some intra-individual variation[13] and this may be a limitation of the usefulness of this marker. Some authors[14] claim that the intact amino-terminal propeptide of type I procollagen (PCINP), a protein set free from the other end of the same procollagen molecule, is a more dynamic marker for bone metabolism than PCICP. According to these authors, it can therefore be recommended that PCINP be used as a marker to reflect the effect of estrogen on bone collagen formation during estrogen replacement therapy. Evidence is now available[15] showing that collagen markers can be a useful tool in predicting osteoporosis and fracture risks, rather than bone mineral density measurements alone. It remains to be shown just how soon after treatment these collagen markers will change, although cross-link excretion has been shown to decrease characteristically after 6 months of treatment.

The end result is that a lack of estrogen present in the postmenopausal years causes this loss of bone mass and clinically results in osteoporosis, with subsequent related osteoporotic fractures of the spine or hip in women. Nowadays, this state of affairs is both preventable and treatable and it should no longer be accepted as a normal process of aging. Health-care physicians must be aware of this and they should strive to try to prevent, or at least to treat, osteoporosis.

SKIN

The skin is one of the largest organs in the body and contains a sizeable proportion of the total body collagen. This organ is composed of a population of cells of diverse embryonic origin, which, under normal conditions, exist side by side in complete harmony, forming a complex mosaic.

Atrophy of the dermis after the menopause is due to a decrease in the dermal skin collagen content. The amounts of hydroxyproline and glycosylated hydroxylysine[16,17] in type I collagen and the number of immature and reducible cross-links decrease with age[18]. To what extent these changes are fundamental to the aging process is still unknown. This decrease is not only arrested, but also reversed, by hormone replacement therapy[19]. There is now strong evidence, as seen from the National Health and Nutrition Examination Survey[3], that estrogen use prevents dry skin and skin wrinkling, thus extending the potential benefits of postmenopausal estrogen therapy to include protection against selected age- and menopause-associated dermatological conditions.

Estrogens have, in fact, been shown to enhance the dermal content of water, glycosaminoglycans and collagen. Both estrogen and androgen receptors have been identified on dermal fibroblasts[20].

Estrogen could increase the rate of collagen production[21] by altering the degree of polymerization of glycosaminoglycans. Estrogens increase the hydroscopic qualities, probably through enhanced synthesis of dermal hyaluronic acid[22,23]. Collagenous fibrils have been found to be less fragmented in the dermis of women treated with estrogens[24].

Studies have been carried out on skin changes in various connective tissue and endocrine disorders. Black[25] and Shuster and colleagues[26] looked at the relationship between skin thickness and skin collagen content in women with systemic sclerosis, those with osteoporosis of mixed etiology and in hirsute women, and found a good correlation between the two. In a small study, Black[25] demonstrated changes in the collagen content and thickness of the skin in osteoporotics (mixed etiology) who were treated with androgens, compared to osteoporotics who had not been on this treatment. Shuster and co-workers found an increase in the skin collagen content in hirsute women, but the increase was not statistically significant[26].

Reports on skin collagen changes with age are conflicting. Shuster and Bottoms[27,28] showed that the best way of expressing skin collagen content was by calculating the collagen content of a skin biopsy per square millimeter of skin surface. This method takes into account the possibility of changes in the total mass of the dermis. Shuster and Bottoms[27,28] reported a reduction in total skin collagen with age, but this was not confirmed by Reed and Hall[29]. Shuster and colleagues[26] found that the amount of collagen present in the skin was at all ages higher in males than in females. Hall and associates[19] confirmed that the skin collagen content was higher in males than in females, but once again could not significantly confirm the decline of skin collagen with age. With increasing age past the menopause, the skin tends to get thinner; this is reversed with adequate estrogen replacement therapy[6]. This was first noted by Albright and colleagues[30] in 1940; they reported that old women with osteoporotic fractures had a higher incidence of thin skin. McConkey and co-workers[31] also showed that osteoporosis was more common in women with transparent skin than in women with thick opaque skin.

The dermal skin thickness itself, composed as it is of connective tissue, including the predominant protein, collagen, as well as elastin (small amounts) and glycoaminoglycans, has also got more than one variable that is affected by a lack of estrogen or its replacement. For example, it has been shown that, over a period of 2 weeks, castrated rats that were given estrogens had a 70% increase in their glycosaminoglycan content[21]. Similar increases in women would lead to skin thickness increases that far outweigh those that would be expected from collagen content increases alone.

Most studies have measured the thickness of dermis, since this is the layer which is mainly composed of connective tissue. Subcutaneous tissue is an added variable and studies using Harpenden's calipers that also include subcutaneous fat have been conflicting[32]. Ultrasound can nowadays be used to measure skin thickness[33]. Ultrasound examination has been used by dermatologists when assessing dermal malignancies. Good reproducibility has been obtained by using high-frequency (22 MHz) ultrasound to determine the thickness of the skin excluding the subcutaneous tissues. Various studies have now shown that skin thickness increases with estrogen replacement therapy. Skin changes and bone changes with estrogen at the menopause are linked together[6,7].

In animals, estrogens appear to alter the vascularization of the skin[34] and a change in the connective tissue of the dermis occurs, as is reflected by increased mucopolysaccharide incorporation, hydroxyproline turnover and alterations in ground substance. In addition to increased dermal turnover of hyaluronic acid, the dermal water content is enhanced with estradiol therapy[23]. Rauramo and Punnonen[35] observed that oral estrogen therapy in castrated women caused thickening of the epidermis for 3 months and this persisted for 6 months.

Punnonen[36], using two different strengths of estrogen in castrated women, showed a statistically significant thickening of the epidermis after 3 months with both strengths, but this thickness persisted only with the lower dose. One-third of the patients on the higher dose started getting significant thinning of the epidermis, possibly because the dosage of the treatment was too strong and was therefore exerting a corticosteroid effect. Other authors were also able to show beneficial skin changes using both topical estradiol[7,37] and estradiol implants[38]. Topical estradiol gel has also been shown to increase skin collagen content, as measured by skin hydroxyproline. Skin blister fluids were assayed and increases in PCICP and PCINP were observed when using the gel.

In comparing a group of patients who had been on estradiol and testosterone implants for 2–10 years with a group of untreated postmenopausal women, it was shown that the treated group had a skin collagen content that was highly significantly greater than in the untreated group. Optimum skin collagen was obtained after 2 years of being on an optimum estrogen regimen. Levels that are too high or too low give lower levels of collagen[39]. The same conclusions were also reported in relation to the epidermis[40].

The decline in skin collagen content after the menopause occurs at a much more rapid rate in the initial postmenopausal years than in the later ones. Approximately 30% of skin collagen is lost in the first 5 years after the menopause[39], with an average decline of 2.1% per postmenopausal year over a period of 20 years. The increase in skin collagen content after 6 months of sex hormone therapy depends on the collagen content at the start of treatment[39]. In women with a low skin collagen content, estrogens are initially of therapeutic and later of prophylactic value, while in those with a mild loss of collagen content in the early menopausal years, estrogens are of prophylactic value only. Thus, a deficiency in skin collagen content can be corrected, but not overcorrected.

Skin collagen content has been shown to have a strong correlation with skin dermal thickness measured radiologically[39]. Using 100 mg subcutaneous estradiol implants, significant increases in skin thickness and metacarpal index occurred over a 1-year period. Most of the increase occurred in the first 6 months.

Brincat and colleagues[37,39] and Castelo-Branco and associates[41] have shown that, following the menopause, skin collagen content and skin thickness are increased in women on estrogen replacement therapy compared to age-matched women on no treatment. Prospective studies have shown that skin thickness, skin collagen and bone mass increase in postmenopausal women who start estrogen replacement therapy. Estrogen has been shown to reduce collagen turnover and improve the quality of collagen[42,43]. When postmenopausal women were treated with topical estrogens[44], it was found that, after treatment for 6 months, elasticity and firmness of the skin had markedly improved and the wrinkle depth and pore sizes had decreased by 61–100%. Furthermore, skin moisture was also increased and the measurement of wrinkles using skin profilometry revealed significant, or even highly significant, decreases in the wrinkles. On immunohistochemistry of the same subjects, significant increases of type III collagen labelling were combined with increased numbers of collagen fibers at the end of the treatment period. This was also confirmed by Creidi and colleagues in their study[45].

The mechanical properties of the skin have been shown to be improved with estrogen replacement therapy in other studies[46,47]. In these studies, the mechanical properties of the skin were defined by ostensibility and elasticity measurements using a computerized device. Computerized measurements of skin deformability and viscoelasticity revealed differences between women on estrogen therapy, postmenopausal women on no treatment and non-menopausal controls. This parallels the changes noted elsewhere with skin collagen. A steep increase in skin extensibility was evidenced during the perimenopause in untreated women. Estrogen replacement therapy appeared to limit the age-related increase in cutaneous extensibility, thereby exerting a preventive effect on skin slackness. Estrogen replacement therapy was found to have no effect on other parameters of skin viscoelasticity. Estrogen replacement therapy has a beneficial effect on some mechanical properties of skin and thus may slow the progress of intrinsic cutaneous aging.

Brincat and co-workers[38,47,48] found significant correlations between the skin (dermal) collagen, skin thickness (measured radiologically) and metacarpal index, both in postmenopausal women who had been on estrogen replacement therapy and in untreated postmenopausal women. The common factor is the connective tissue present in all three sites. These findings were irrespective of the woman's age, number of years since the menopause, original skin thickness and metacarpal index.

Attempts to identify the correct value of skin thickness that could be used to screen for menopausal osteoporosis have been under way for some time[49].

CAROTID ARTERIES

The cardioprotective effect of hormone replacement therapy has been proved over the years[50]. This has been attributed to the favorable serum lipoprotein profile brought about by this treatment in postmenopausal women[51]. Only a 20–25% reduction in coronary artery plaque formation can, however, be thus accounted for[52]; other mechanisms of cardioprevention are therefore present. One such mechanism could be due to postmenopausal connective tissue changes which mimic those in skin and bone. Using high frequency ultrasound, our group looked at the differences in the layers of one of the major blood vessels, the carotid artery. One study investigated differences in the externa and media of the carotid artery in a group of postmenopausal women on oral estrogen replacement therapy, in another group of women being treated with estradiol implants and in an untreated group of postmenopausal women; the intima was also assessed. The results showed that the media, the layer containing the greatest amount of collagen, was thicker in both of the estrogen-treated groups than in the untreated group. The intima of the untreated group was also shown to be significantly thicker than that of the group on estrogen replacement therapy (Figure 4). This signifies that there was less athersclerotic plaque in the treated than in the untreated group. However, in women on a higher dose of estrogen (i.e. those being treated with estradiol implants), the intima was as thick as in the untreated group. This was postulated as being due to the collagen portion of the intima following the media and increasing in size at the expense of thinning of the athersclerotic plaque as this is lost[53, 54]. It has thus been suggested that these changes are brought about by estrogens. If these arterial changes induced by hormone replacement therapy also occur in the coronary arteries,

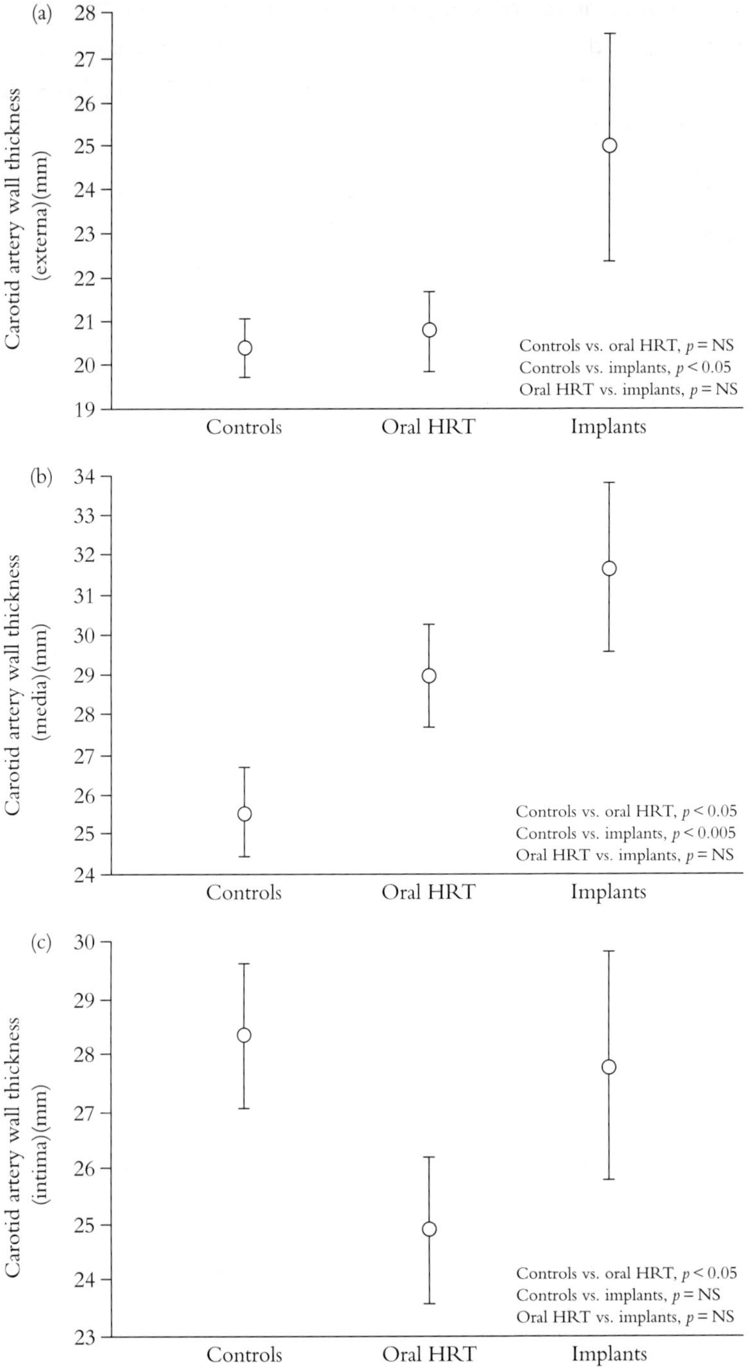

Figure 4 Plots (mean ± SE) of carotid artery wall thickness ((a), externa; (b), media; (c), intima) in postmenopausal women on no treatment (n = 51), oral hormone replacement therapy (HRT) (n = 46) and estradiol implants (n = 32)

and some suggestion of this has been made, then these changes may partially explain the cardioprotective effect that this treatment has on postmenopausal women.

CONCLUSION

The connective tissue component in the body represents a complex mass of cells and extracellular matrix that are intimately related to each other and provide a milieu in which all the other cells are able to perform their functions and relate to each other. The collagen components themselves, so vitally important to the organism, undergo measurable changes with estrogen deprivation, but happily this is preventable and to a degree replaceable with appropriate estrogen therapy. Early evidence suggests that selective estrogen receptor modulators (SERMs) have the same effect and raloxifine chloride has been shown to have the same effect on estrogen markers as estrogens.

In conclusion, sex steroids play a vital role in the integrity of the tissues of an individual and this constitutes yet another strong argument for long-term hormone replacement therapy or treatment with SERMs.

REFERENCES

1. Murry RK, Keeley FW. The extracellular matrix. In Murray RK, Granner DK, Mayes PA, Rodwell VW, eds. *Harper's Biochemistry*, 24th edn. London: Appleton and Lange, 1996: 667–85
2. Punnonen R, Vilska S, Rauramo L. Skinfold thickness and long-term post-menopausal hormone therapy. *Maturitas* 1984;5:259–62
3. Dunn LB, Damesyn M, Moore AA, Reuben DB, Greendale GA. Does estrogen prevent skin aging? Results from the First National Health and Nutrition Examination Survey (NHANESI). *Arch Dermatol* 1997;133:339–42
4. Schmidt JB, Binder M, Demschik G, Bieglmayer C, Reiner A. Treatment of skin aging with topical estrogens. *Int J Dermatol* 1996;35:669–74
5. The Writing Group for the PEPI trial. Effects of hormone therapy on bone mineral density: results from the postmenopausal estrogen/progestin intervention (PEPI) trial. *J Am Med Assoc* 1996;276:1389–96
6. Brincat M, Moniz CR, Kabalan S, *et al.* Decline in skin collagen content and metacarpal index after the menopause and its prevention with sex hormone replacement. *Br J Obstet Gynaecol* 1987;94:126–9
7. Brincat M, Kabalan S, Studd JWW, *et al.* A study of the relationship of skin collagen content, skin thickness and bone mass in the postmenopausal woman. *Obstet Gynecol* 1987;70: 840–5
8. Gordan GS. Prevention of bone loss and fractures in women. *Maturitas* 1984;6:225–42

9. Brincat M, Galea R, Muscat Baron Y. A screening model for osteoporosis using dermal skin thickness and bone densitometry. In Wren BG, ed. *Progress in the Management of the Menopause*. Carnforth, UK: Parthenon Publishing, 1996:175–8
10. Väänänen HK, Härkönen PL. Estrogen and bone metabolism. *Maturitas* 1996;23 (Suppl 10):S65–9
11. Schneider DL, Barrett Connor EL, Morton DJ. Timing of postmenopausal estrogen for optimal bone mineral density. The Rancho Bernardo Study. *J Am Med Assoc* 1997;277: 543–7
12. Brincat M, Galea R, Muscat Baron Y, Xuereb A. Changes in bone collagen markers and in bone density in hormone treated and untreated postmenopausal women. *Maturitas* 1997;27:171–7
13. Ginty F, Flynn A, Cashman K. Inter and intra-individual variations in urinary excretion of pyridinium crosslinks of collagen in healthy young adults. *Eur J Clin Nutr* 1998;52:71–3
14. Suvanto Luukkonen E, Risteli L, Sundström H, Penttinen J, Kauppila A, Risteli J. Comparison of three serum assays for bone collagen formation during postmenopausal estrogen–progestin therapy. *Clin Chim Acta* 1997;266:105–16
15. Melton LJ III, Khosla S, Atkinson EJ, O'Fallon WM, Riggs BL. Relationship of bone turnover to bone density and fractures. *J Bone Miner Res* 1997;12:1083–91
16. Barnes MJ, Constable BJ, Morton LF, *et al.* Age-related variations in hydroxylation of lysine and proline on collagen. *Biochem J* 1974;139:461–8
17. Murai A, Miyahara T, Shiozawa S. Age-related variations in glycosylation of hydroxy-proline in human and rat skin collagens. *Biochim Biophys Acta* 1975;404:345–8
18. Risteli J, Kivirikko KI. Intracellular enzymes of collagen biosynthesis in rat liver as a function of age and in hepatic injury induced by dimethylnitrosamine: changes in prolyl hydroxylase, lysyl hydroxylase, collagen galactosyltransferase and collagen glucosyltransferase activities. *Biochem J* 1976;158:361–7
19. Hall DA, Reed FB, Noki G, Vince JD. The relative effects of age and corticosteroid therapy on the collagen profiles of dermis from subjects with rheumatoid arthritis. *Age Ageing* 1974;3:15–22
20. Stumpf WE, Sur M, Joshi SE. Estrogen target cells in the skin. *Experimentia* 1976;30:196
21. Boucek RJ, Noble NL, Woessner JF Jr. Properties of fibroblasts. In Page IH, ed. *Connective Tissue Thrombosis and Atherosclerosis*. New York: Academic Press, 1959:193–211
22. Danforth DN, Vies A, Breen M, Weinstein HG, Buckingham JC, Manalo P. The effect of pregnancy and labour on the human cervix: changes in collagen, glycoproteins and glucosaminoglycans. *Am J Obstet Gynecol* 1974;120:641–51
23. Grosman N, Hindberg E, Schen J. The effect of oestrogenic treatment on the acid mucopolysaccharide pattern in skin of mice. *Acta Pharmacol Toxicol* 1971;30:458–64
24. Goldzieher MA. The effects of oestrogens on the senile skin. *J Gerontol* 1946;1:196
25. Black MM. A modified radiographic method for measuring skin thickness. *Br J Dermatol* 1969;1:661
26. Shuster J, Black MM, McVitie E. The influence of age and sex on skin thickness, skin collagen and density. *Br J Dermatol* 1975;93:639
27. Shuster S, Bottoms E. Senile degeneration of skin collagen. *Clin Sci* 1963;25:487–91
28. Shuster S, Bottoms E. Effect of ultraviolet light on skin collagen. *Mature* 1963;199:192–3

29. Reed VB, Hall DA. In Frische R, Hartmann F, eds. *Connective Tissues – Biochemistry and Pathophysiology*. Berlin: Spinger Verlag, 1974:290
30. Albright F, Bloomberg E, Smith PH. Postmenopausal osteoporosis. *Tram Assoc Am Phys* 1940;55:298–305
31. McConkey B, Fraser GR, Bligh AS, Whitely M. Transparent skin and osteoporosis, *Lancet* 1963;1:693–5
32. Varila E, Rantala I, Ikarinem A, *et al.* The effect of topical oestriol on skin collagen of postmenopausal women. *Br J Obstet Gynaecol* 1995;102:985–9
33. Tan CY, Stratham B, Marks R, Payne PA. Skin thickness measurements by pulsed ultrasound: its reproducibility, validation and variability. *Br J Dermatol* 1994;96:1392–4
34. Goodrich SM, Wood JE. The effect of oestradiol 17β on peripheral venous distensibility and velocity of venous blood flow. *Am J Obstet Gynecol* 1966;96:407–12
35. Rauramo, L, Punnonen R. Wirking einer oralen estrogentherapie mit oestriolsuccinat auf die haut hastierter. *Frauen Haut Gerchluts Kr* 1969;44:463–70
36. Punnonen R. Effect of castration and peroral therapy on skin. *Acta Obstet Gynaecol Scand* 1973;21(Suppl):1–4
37. Brincat M, Moniz CJ, Studd JWW, *et al.* Long term effects of the menopause and sex hormones on skin thickness. *Br J Obstet Gynaecol* 1985;92:256–9
38. Brincat M, Moniz CJ, Kabalan S, *et al.* Decline in skin collagen content and metacarpal index after the menopause and its prevention with sex hormone replacement. *Br J Obstet Gynaecol* 1987;94:126–9
39. Brincat M, Moniz CF, Studd JWW, *et al.* Sex hormones and skin collagen content in postmenopausal women. *Br Med J* 1983;287:1337–8
40. Shahrad P, Marks RA. Pharmacological effect of oestrone on human epidermis. *Br J Dermatol* 1977;97:383–6
41. Castelo-Branco C, Duran M, Gonzalez-Merlo J. Skin collagen changes related to age and hormone replacement therapy. *Maturitas* 1992;15:113–19
42. Castelo-Barcia C, Pons F, Gratacos E, Fortuny A, Panrell JA, Gonzalez Merlo J. Relationship between skin collagen and bone changes during ageing. *Maturitas* 1994;18:199–206
43. Holland EFN, Studd JWW, Mansell JP, Leather AT, Bailey AJ. Changes in collagen composition and cross-links in bone and skin of osteoporotic postmenopausal women treated with percutaneous estradiol implants. *Obstet Gynecol* 1994;83:180–3
44. Schmidt JB, Binder M, Demschik G, Bieglmayer C, Reiner A. Treatment of skin aging with topical estrogens. *Int J Dermatol* 1996;35:669–74
45. Creidi P, Faivre B, Agache P, Richard E, Haudiquet V, Sauvanet JP. Effect of a conjugated oestrogen (Premarin) cream on ageing facial skin. A comparative study with a placebo cream. *Maturitas* 1994;19:211–23
46. Pverard GE, Letawe L, Dowlati A, Pierard-Franchimant L. Effect of hormone replacement therapy for menopause on the mechanical properties of skin. *J Am Soc* 1995;43: 662–4
47. Brincat M, Studd JWW, Moniz CF, Parsons V, Darby AJ. Skin thickness and skin collagen mimic an index of osteoporosis in the postmenopausal woman. In Christiansen C, *et al.*, eds. *Osteoporosis. Proceedings of the Copenhagen International Symposium on Osteoporosis*. 1984; 1:353–5

48. Brincat M, Studd JWW, Moniz CF, Parsons V, Darby AJ. Skin thickness measurment. A simple screening method for determining patients at risk of postmenopausal osteoporosis. In Christiansen C, *et al.*, eds. *Osteoporosis. Proceedings of the Copenhagen International Symposium on Osteoporosis*. 1984;1:323–6
49. Brincat M, Galea R, Muscat Baron Y. A screening model for osteoporosis using dermal skin thickness and bone densitometry. In Wren BG, ed. *Progress in Management of the Menopause*. Carnforth, UK: Parthenon Publishing, 1997:175–8
50. Stampfer MJ, Colditz GA, Willem WC, *et al.* Postmenopausal oestrogen therapy and cardiovascular disease. Ten year follow-up from The Nurses' Health Study. *N Engl J Med* 1991;325:756–62
51. PEPI Trial Writing Group. Effects of estrogen and estrogen/progesterone regimens on heart disease risk factors in postmenopausal women. The postmenopausal estrogen/progestogen intervention (PEPI) trial. *J Am Med Assoc* 1995;273:199–208
52. Adams MR, Kaplan JR, Mauck SB. Inhibition of coronary artery atherosclerosis by 17β-Estradiolin ovariectomised monkeys: lack of an effect of added progesterone. *Atherosclerosis* 1990;10:1051–7
53. Muscat Baron Y, Brincat M, Galea R. Carotid artery wall thickness in women treated with hormone replacement therapy. *Maturitas* 1997;27:47–53
54. Muscat Baron Y, Galea R, Brincat M. Carotid artery wall changes in estrogen treated and untreated postmenopausal women. *Obstet Gynecol* 1998;91:1982–6

9

Continuous combined HRT

D. W. Sturdee

INTRODUCTION

While the benefits of hormone replacement therapy (HRT) are becoming increasingly well established and accepted, it is self-evident that women will not achieve such effects if they do not continue with HRT for long enough. Compliance or continuance is surprisingly poor, with around 25% of women stopping therapy within 6 months and few continuing for more than 1 or 2 years. The main reasons for discontinuing HRT include cyclical, period-type bleeding, fear of cancer, unacceptable or unexpected side-effects, such as breast tenderness, and premenstrual syndrome-type symptoms[1].

Sequential regimens of HRT are intended to mimic the ovarian cycle, whereas continuous combined therapy (CCT) provides the same dose of estrogen and progestogen every day without a break so that there is no cycle. The continuous daily progestogen is the fundamental difference between these regimens, which has been especially pioneered in Scandinavia and Europe[2–5]. With further evidence of the benefits, there are more proprietary regimens becoming available and the use of CCT is increasing.

TREATMENT COMBINATION OPTIONS

Initial reports on CCT were with oral regimens, either in a fixed-dose combination, such as estradiol 2 mg with norethisterone acetate 1 mg[2,3], or with varying-dose combinations, particularly of the progestogen to obtain optimum prevention of bleeding[4]. With the rapid expansion in the number of hormone preparations and routes of administration of estrogen and progestogen, there are now many different options for providing CCT (Table 1). In the UK there are seven fixed-dose proprietary preparations (Table 2) and the gonadomimetic tibolone, which has similar effects to CCT[6]. The

Table 1 Options for routes of administration of estrogen and progestogen in continuous combined regimens. Routes in brackets are under development or not yet licensed for this purpose in the UK

Estrogen	*Progestogen*
Tablet	Tablet
Skin patch or gel	Skin patch
Subcutaneous pellet implant	Vaginal gel
(Vaginal ring)	Suppository
(Nasal spray)	(Intrauterine device)

Table 2 Period-free therapy

Type	*Brand®*	*Estrogen*	*Progestogen*	*Formulation*
Continuous combined therapy	Climesse (Merigest)*	estradiol 2 mg	norethisterone 0.7 mg	tablets
Continuous combined therapy	Kliofem (Kliogest)*	estradiol 2 mg	norethisterone 1 mg	tablets
Continuous combined therapy	Kliovance (Activelle)*	estradiol 1 mg	norethisterone 0.5 mg	tablets
Continuous combined therapy	Elleste duet conti (Femanor/ Estratab)*	estradiol 2 mg	norethisterone 1 mg	tablets
Continuous combined therapy	Nuvelle continuous	estradiol 2 mg	norethisterone 1 mg	tablets
Continuous combined therapy	Premique (Premelle)*	CEE 0.625 mg	MPA 5 mg	tablets
Continuous combined therapy	Evorel conti (Systen conti)*	estradiol 50 μg	norethisterone 170 μg	patches
Gonadomimetic	Livial (Liviel/ Bottin)*	tibolone 2.5 mg		tablets

*Brand names in some countries other than UK. CEE, conjugated equine estrogens; MPA, medroxyprogesterone acetate

levonorgestrel-releasing intrauterine device Mirena®, which is at present only licensed in the UK for contraception, will produce an atrophic endometrium and has been used for CCT together with either oral or transdermal estrogen[7,8].

BLEEDING AND THE ENDOMETRIUM

Although the main aim of CCT is to avoid cyclical bleeding, all studies of CCT have found a particularly high incidence of bleeds in the first 3 months, varying from 50 to 80%. This occurs more often in women who are within 1 year of the menopause, rather than in postmenopausal women, probably due to some residual ovarian activity. The European Consensus Development Conference in 1996 concluded that it is possible to achieve a bleed-free regimen in 60–75% of women who are at least 1 year postmenopause[9].

The bleeds are usually light and are often only intermittent spotting. With time it becomes less, so that few women are bleeding after 12 months[3,4,10,11]. The development of low-dose combinations with 1 mg estradiol or equivalent may cause less bleeding[12,13]. The gonadomimetic hormone tibolone is specifically converted in the endometrium to its Δ4-metabolite, which has no estrogenic activity, so the endometrium is not stimulated. One comparative study of tibolone with CCT does suggest a lower incidence of bleeding or spotting[14].

Several studies have confirmed that an atrophic endometrium is achieved with CCT in 90–100% of women, even after only 3 months of treatment, with daily doses of progestogen as low as 0.35 mg norethisterone acetate[4] or 2.5 mg medroxyprogesterone acetate (MPA)[13,15]. After 1 year of treatment with conjugated equine estrogens 0.625 mg and MPA 2.5 mg or 5.0 mg daily, Woodruff and Pickar[15] found endometrial hyperplasia without atypia in less than 1%, which is lower than the background rate in postmenopausal women. Furthermore, Wells[16] reported that, in women who had complex endometrial hyperplasia while taking standard sequential estrogen/progestogen regimens, the endometrium became normal after 9 months of CCT. A recent study from Sweden has found not only an increased risk of endometrial cancer with long-term standard sequential HRT regimens, but a significantly reduced incidence with CCT[17]. After 5 or more years of CCT use, the odds ratio for developing endometrial cancer was 0.2 (95% confidence interval 0.1–0.8).

There have been two reports of endometrial cancer in women taking CCT; in all of the cases there were predisposing factors such as previous atypical endometrial hyperplasia or prolonged use of unopposed estrogen therapy[18,19]. There are no reports of endometrial cancer developing from a normal endometrium in women who are taking CCT. All these data suggest that the continuous progestogen in CCT provides better protection of the endometrium, which is particularly important for long-term therapy.

CARDIOVASCULAR DISEASE RISK FACTORS

The increasing prevalence of cardiovascular disease in postmenopausal women is associated with an unfavorable change in the blood lipid profile after the menopause, and in particular a rise in total cholesterol. Estrogen replacement therapy causes a favorable change in the lipid profile, and this may contribute up to 30% of the total benefit in reducing cardiovascular disease risk[20]. Progestogen derivatives of 19-nortestosterone have been shown to affect adversely the beneficial estrogenic effect on serum lipoproteins[21], and mainly for this reason there has been some reluctance to accept that CCT could be a suitable regimen for long-term HRT. However, several studies with different combinations of estrogen and progestogen have demonstrated a significant reduction in total cholesterol and in low density lipoprotein (LDL) cholesterol, with little difference between them[5,20,22]. The main effect of progestogens seems to be to blunt the rise of high density lipoprotein (HDL) cholesterol that is induced by estrogen alone, but the reduction of the LDL fraction may be greater and the overall effect is therefore considered to be beneficial. Raised serum triglyceride is also an independent risk factor for coronary heart disease (CHD), and this tends to rise after the menopause and to be increased further by oral estrogen. Studies of CCT with MPA have shown variable effects (either little change or a slight increase), although norethisterone can reduce the levels of triglyceride significantly[5,22,23].

There is no evidence that CCT alters systolic or diastolic blood pressure or causes weight gain[5,22].

There are many long-term observational studies looking at the effects of HRT on cardiovascular disease, but none of them have contained data on CCT. However, a recently reported randomized placebo-controlled secondary prevention (HERS) study assessed the effect of CCT with conjugated equine estrogens 0.625 mg and MPA 2.5 mg daily on the risk of myocardial infarction[24]. The women had a mean age of 67 years and proven coronary artery disease, and were studied for just over 4 years. Overall, there were no significant differences between the placebo and CCT groups in the occurrence of non-fatal myocardial infarction, although the incidence was significantly greater in the treatment group during the first year. Subsequently, there were fewer events in years 4 and 5, producing a statistically significant favorable time trend. Analysis of the time trend suggested a possible late benefit of treatment, and it is very regrettable that the study was not continued for a further 6–12 months, which might have demonstrated a definite benefit from CCT. This study also found a significant excess risk of venous thrombosis in the CCT users (relative hazard 2.9, 95% confidence interval 1.50–5.58), which is similar to other reports for HRT[25]. The HERS study has received much critical analysis, and in particular it is not clear what relevance the findings have for postmenopausal women who do not have coronary artery disease. Furthermore, there are no observational data on CHD risk in other postmenopausal women taking this particular regimen of CCT. A recent report on CCT with the same combination of conjugated equine estrogens and MPA as in the HERS study found no unfavorable effects on either coagulation factors or fibrinolytic components. In addition, unopposed conjugated equine estrogens caused an increase in factor VII, which was corrected by the addition of MPA[26].

Current use of HRT is thought to provide an approximately 50% reduction in CHD risk[20], but the long-term effects will not be established until larger and more powerful prospective randomized controlled trials using different CCT regimens are completed. These include a study by the Women's Health Initiative (WHI) in the United States, which will report in 2005, and the Medical Research Council's Women's International Study of long Duration Oestrogen after Menopause (WISDOM) in Europe, which will be complete in 2012[27].

OSTEOPOROSIS

The prevention of bone loss by estrogen and combined sequential regimens of HRT is well established. Some progestogens, particularly norethisterone, can have an independent effect in preventing bone loss in postmenopausal women[28]. When used in CCT regimens, there may be an additive effect to that of estrogen, thus increasing the benefits for bone protection and the initial replacement of bone loss[5]. With long-term use, the increase in lumbar vertebral bone mineral density may be greater with CCT than with sequential regimens[29].

BREAST CANCER

None of the various reports on HRT and breast cancer have any or sufficient data on CCT regimens to indicate whether there is any difference in the risk between unopposed estrogen and sequential estrogen/progestogen regimens. The HERS study was not powerful enough, but hopefully the other ongoing studies will provide satisfactory data on this aspect as well as for cardiovascular disease. It is unlikely that the continuous progestogen will alter the overall slightly increased risk with long-term use after the menopause, and women should be counselled accordingly.

COMPLIANCE

CCT is most suitable for women who are at least 1 year postmenopause, when symptom control is less important than long-term benefits, although flushes and sweats are relieved by CCT[12,13]. Side-effects of sequential estrogen/progestogen HRT are often due to the progestogen component and are similar to those of the premenstrual syndrome[1]. Each month these problems may be triggered by the introduction of the 10–12-day phase of progestogen. With CCT there is no cycle or change in hormone levels, so that premenstrual syndrome-type side-effects seem to be less of a problem. However, the continuous progestogen may still cause breast tenderness and abdominal bloating, and a lower dose may be more satisfactory if these problems do not resolve after the initial weeks of treatment[12]. The main advantage of CCT, however, should be the absence of period-type bleeds, and this does improve compliance compared to the monthly sequential regimens[30].

FUTURE

The future will see more lower dose combinations that should further improve compliance and will be particularly suitable for older postmenopausal women who do not need the same dose as women around the time of the menopause. Development of intrauterine progestogen-releasing devices, vaginal rings, nasal sprays and other transdermal systems will provide further options and greater long-term acceptability.

Treatment strategies for long-term therapy are changing because of the increased risk of breast cancer with long-term HRT use and evidence that the benefits on bone and cardiovascular protection are soon lost on cessation of treatment. Treatment for several years following the menopause will provide symptom relief and some bone and heart protection, but the main risks of CHD and osteoporotic fractures are in women over the age of 70. Starting or resuming HRT over the age of 60 with a low-dose CCT regimen seems to be a good option.

REFERENCES

1. MacLennan AH, MacLennan A, O'Neill S, Kirkgard Y, Wenzel SR, Chamber HM. Oestrogen and cyclical progestogen in postmenopausal hormone replacement therapy. *Med J Aust* 1992;157:167–70
2. Staland B. Continuous treatment with a combination of estrogen and gestagen – a way of avoiding endometrial stimulation. *Acta Obstet Gynaecol Scand* 1982;130(Suppl):29–35
3. Mattsson LÅ. Cullberg G, Samsioe G. Evaluation of a continuous combined oestrogen/progestogen regimen for climacteric complaints. *Maturitas* 1982;4:95–102
4. Magos A, Brincat M, Studd JWW, Wardle P, Schlesinger P, O'Dowd T. Amenorrhoea and endometrial atrophy with continuous oral estrogens and progestin therapy in post-menopausal women. *Obstet Gynecol* 1985;65:496–9
5. Christiansen C, Riis BJ. 17β-Estradiol and continuous norethisterone: a unique treatment for established osteoporosis in elderly women. *J Clin Endocrinol Metab* 1990;71:836–41

6. Moore RA. Livial: a review of clinical studies. *Br J Obstet Gynaecol* 1999;106(Suppl 19):1–21
7. Andersson K, Mattsson L-Å, Rybo G, Stadberg G. Intrauterine release of levonorgestrel – a new way of adding progestogen in hormone replacement therapy. *Obstet Gynecol* 1992;79:963–7
8. Randaskoski TH, Lahti EI, Kauppila AJ. Transdermal estrogen with a levonorgestrel-releasing intrauterine device for climacteric complaints; clinical and endometrial responses. *Am J Obstet Gynecol* 1995;172:114–19
9. Birkhäuser M, Rosenbaum H. *Menopause – European Consensus Development Conference*. Paris: Editions Eska, 1996:29
10. Pickar JH, Bottiglioni F, Archer DF. Amenorrhea frequency with continuous combined hormone replacement therapy: a retrospective analysis. *Climacteric* 1998;1:130–6
11. Udoff L, Langenberg P, Adaski EY. Combined continuous hormone replacement therapy: a critical review. *Obstet Gynecol* 1995;86:306–16
12. Baerug U, Winge T, Nordland G, *et al*. Do combinations of 1 mg estradiol and low doses of NETA effectively control menopausal symptoms? *Climacteric* 1998;1:219–28
13. Nand SL, Webster MA, Baber R, O'Connor V. Amenorrhea was achieved in most women after 6 months of continuous combined hormone replacement therapy, even with low-dose progesterone. *Obstet Gynecol* 1998;91:678–84
14. Hammar M, Christau S, Nathorst-Böös J, Rud T, Garre K. A double blind, randomised trial comparing the effects of tibolone and continuous combined hormone replacement therapy in postmenopausal women with menopausal symptoms. *Br J Obstet Gynaecol* 1998;105:904–11
15. Woodruff JD, Pickar JH. Incidence of endometrial hyperplasia in postmenopausal women taking conjugated estrogens (Premarin) with medroxyprogesterone acetate or conjugated estrogens alone. *Am J Obstet Gynecol* 1994;170:1213–23
16. Wells M. Endometrial response to continuous combined HRT. Presented at the *8th International Congress on the Menopause*, Sydney, Australia, 1996:abstr 539
17. Weiderpass E, Adani H-O, Baron JA, *et al*. Risk of endometrial cancer following estrogen replacement with and without progestins. *J Natl Cancer Inst* 1999;91:1131–7
18. Leather AT, Savvas M, Studd JWW. Endometrial histology and bleeding patterns after 8 years of continuous combined estrogen and progestogen therapy in postmenopausal women. *Obstet Gynecol* 1991;78:1008–10
19. Comerci JT, Fields AL, Runowicz CD, Goldberg GL. Continuous low-dose combined hormone replacement therapy and the risk of endometrial cancer. *Gynecol Oncol* 1997;64: 425–30
20. Barrett-Connor E, Grady D. Hormone replacement therapy, heart disease and other considerations. *Annu Rev Public Health* 1998;19:55–72
21. Hirvonen E, Mälkönen M, Manninen V. Effects of different progestogens on lipoproteins during postmenopausal replacement therapy. *N Engl J Med* 1991;304:560–3
22. The Writing Group for the PEPI trial. Effects of estrogen or estrogen/progestin regimens on heart disease risk factors in postmenopausal women: the Postmenopausal Estrogen/ Progestin Interventions (PEPI) trial. *J Am Med Assoc* 1995;273:199–208

23. Speroff L, Rowan J, Symons J, Genaut H, Wilborn W. The comparative effect on bone density, endometrium and lipids of continuous hormones as replacement therapy (CHART study): a randomised controlled trial. *J Am Med Assoc* 1996;276:1397–403
24. Hulley S, Grady D, Bush T, *et al.* Randomised trial of estrogen plus progestin for secondary prevention of coronary heart disease in postmenopausal women. *J Am Med Assoc* 1998;280:605–12
25. Daly E, Vessey MP, Hawkins MM, *et al.* Risk of venous thromboembolism in users of hormone replacement therapy. *Lancet* 1996;348:977–80
26. Nozaki M, Ogata R, Koera K, Hashimoto K, Nakamo H. Changes in coagulation factors and fibrinolytic components of postmenopausal women receiving continuous hormone replacement therapy. *Climacteric* 1999;2:124–30
27. Meade TW. HERS and its aftermath [Editorial]. *Climacteric* 1999;2:2–5
28. Abdalla HI, Hart DM, Lindsay R, Leggate I, Hooke A. Prevention of bone mineral loss in postmenopausal women by norethisterone. *Obstet Gynecol* 1985;66:789–92
29. Eiken P, Kolthoff N, Pors Nielsen S. Effect of 10 years' hormone replacement therapy on bone mineral content in postmenopausal women. *Bone* 1996;19(Suppl):191S–3S
30. Dören M, Reuther C, Minne HW, Schneider HPG. Superior compliance and efficacy of continuous combined oral estrogen/progestogen replacement therapy in postmenopausal women. *Am J Obstet Gynecol* 1995;173:1446–51

Gynaecological malignancies

10

ART and gynaecological malignancies

P. N. Barri, M. Izquierdo and B. Coroleu

INTRODUCTION

The etiology of many gynaecological cancers is, even today, poorly understood. It is known that women who have not had children run a higher risk of cancer of the breast, of the ovary and of the endometrium[1,2], a close relationship having been established between the age of the first birth and the risk of cancer of the breast[3,4].

Although the greater risk of gynaecological cancer in childless women appears to be due to their involuntary infertility and the consequent absence of known protection factors such as multiparity and lactation, it is incumbent upon us to deepen our knowledge of the risks additional to those to which involuntarily infertile patients may be subjected.

Present-day assisted reproduction techniques (ART), with their usual protocols of stimulation of follicular development by means of drugs such as clomiphene citrate and the gonadotropins, have been suggested as possible additional risk factors in infertile patients with respect to cancer of the breast, ovary and endometrium[5–10].

PROTECTION AND RISK FACTORS

Numerous publications[1,2,11] agree that factors such as early motherhood, multiparity and breastfeeding have a protective effect against any gynaecological cancer. Patients who have taken anovulatory drugs for a period of time greater than 3 years will have additional protection against ovarian cancer[12,13].

Bearing in mind that gynecological cancer tends to be a multifactorial disease, it is not possible to talk of isolated factors but rather of groups of risk factors, which we could classify in three categories: genetic, hormonal and environmental.

Genetic factors

Ovarian cancer can be considered as an autosomal dominant disease. If there is a grade I family history, the risk of the disease developing is 50%. In these cases, chromosome deletions and allele loss have been described. The subsequent loss of genes of tumoral suppression would result in a greater risk of cancer.

There is evidence of breast and ovarian cancer in families with the presence in a locus on chromosome 17 of the *BRCA-1* gene, the gene of family predisposition to breast and ovarian cancer. Another variety is the presence in a locus on chromosome 13 of the *BRCA-2* gene, which would predispose to breast cancer, but which can cause breast cancer in men.

Now there is knowledge of the LYNCH-II syndrome, in which there are alterations in the short arm of chromosome 2, which involve the loss of DNA repairing genes. The syndrome can manifest itself in forms of family cancer in various locations (colon, stomach, ovary, endometrium and breast)[11].

Hormonal factors

Evidence that a protective effect against gynaecological cancer results from ovulatory interruption, for reasons such as the taking of anovulatory drugs, pregnancy and lactation, confirms the relationship between the hormonal environment and the risk of cancer.

There is controversy surrounding the risk which may be involved in hypergonadotropic states secondary to ovulation induction treatments, especially for breast and endometrial cancer. Controversy surrounds the idea that the majority of epithelial tumors of the ovary are insensitive to gonadotropins because they do not always have binding sites for gonadotropins.

Likewise, there is knowledge of the risk for breast or endometrial cancer, but not for ovarian cancer, associated with a hyperestrogenic environment that is not well balanced with gestagens, as in some protocols of hormone replacement therapy.

Environmental factors

There are data in the literature that suggest a greater incidence of gynecological cancer in industrialized countries than in underdeveloped countries. This is probably due to the higher birth rates and levels of breastfeeding common in the countries of the Third World. There are also factors that have been associated with a greater risk of ovarian cancer, such as talcum powder and excessive consumption of animal fat and whole milk.

DATA FROM THE LITERATURE

Ovarian cancer

Ever since the classic work of Fathalla in 1971[14], which attributed a potential risk of cancer to continued ovarian stimulation with his theory of 'unceasing ovulation', few publications have appeared concerning the protective or risk effect that anovulatory drugs[12,13,15] or fertility treatments had on ovarian cancer[5,7]. Nonetheless, several articles have appeared in recent years which consider the conclusions of the Collaborative Ovarian Cancer Group after evaluating 12 American studies on 2197 white women with ovarian cancer against a control group consisting of 4144 white women[8,9,16]. The final message of their meta-analysis was that the use of ovulation-inducing drugs could increase three-fold the later risk of developing ovarian cancer. These results were quickly contested by the Food and Drug Administration[17], the American Fertility Society[18], the International Federation of Fertility Societies[19], the National Cancer Institute[20] and Stanford University Medical Center[21]. Likewise, various authors individually presented their criticisms of Whittemore's work[1,2,22,23]. The majority of the publications agree in pointing out that the major errors in Whittemore's work are:

(1) It does not distinguish between patients who were ovulating and those who were not.

(2) It does not differentiate between the various ovulation-inducing drugs, the doses used, or the number of treatment cycles.

(3) The confidence intervals were wide, owing to the small numbers of exposed cases and controls.

(4) Only three out of 12 studies contained information about the patients' fertility.

(5) There was skewing in the selection of patients, since many patients were not interviewed.

(6) A significant diagnostic skewing existed, since the majority of the cases were based on differing diagnostic criteria of the tumoral stages.

(7) There was skewing in the selection of the percentage of infertile women for the control group.

(8) Another aspect worthy of consideration is the value of the classic affirmation that ovarian cancer is more common in the right ovary because ovulation is also more frequent in the right ovary[24]. However, we[25] have reviewed 293 cases of epithelial ovarian cancer without finding differences between its location in one ovary or the other. Nor could we find evidence after 156 spontaneous *in vitro* fertilization (IVF) cycles of a greater incidence of ovulation in the right ovary. All this leads us to question seriously the possible relationship which may exist between the ovulating ovary and the later development of epithelial ovarian cancer.

An interesting study of the risk of ovarian cancer among the population of infertile women[26] establishes the potential risk which would be associated with long-term treatment with clomiphene citrate. These authors have analyzed the risk of ovarian cancer in a population of 3837 infertile patients followed up during the period 1974–85. In the study there are 11 cases of malignant ovarian tumor, compared with the 4.4 which would have been expected from the characteristics of the studied population. Clomiphene citrate was the inducing drug administered to nine of the 11 patients who developed ovarian cancer; it is also relevant that five of these nine patients with ovarian cancer had taken clomiphene for 12 or more months, whereas the patients who took the drug for less than 1 year did not show any higher risk for ovarian cancer.

Other studies cover the appearance of ovarian tumors in infertile patients undergoing repeated treatment with ovulatory stimulation[27–29].

There are published cases of two infertile patients undergoing unilateral adnexectomy for a borderline ovarian tumor, with normality in the contralateral ovary, and later treatment with ovarian stimulation for IVF at 3 and 6 months after surgery, which resulted in pregnancy in one of the patients[30].

In Italy, the incidence of ovarian cancer and its relationship with fertility treatment has been followed up in four different regions[31]. This study covers 195 epithelial ovarian cancers and compares them with a control group consisting of 1339 patients without cancer. The intake of ovulation-inducing drugs was less common in the group of patients with ovarian cancer than in the control group (odds ratio 0.7, 95% confidence interval (CI) 0.2–3.3).

Furthermore, over the period 1925–61, a higher cancer mortality rate could not be demonstrated in a group of patients who received radiotherapy in the pituitary gland and ovaries to stimulate ovulation[32].

Detailed analysis of the majority of these studies does not allow the affirmation of a clear causal relationship between infertility treatment and later development of ovarian cancer. Multicenter studies are needed, with long-term follow-up of the patients who underwent ovarian stimulation in assisted reproduction techniques[10].

BREAST CANCER

Breast cancer has also been seen to be related to the previous administration of ovulation-inducing treatment. Sixteen cases of breast cancer have been found among 950 infertile patients treated with ovarian stimulation protocols, who were followed up for 10 years. The authors described an excessive estrogen level, which was not compensated by the low progesterone levels usual in these patients, and demonstrated that 13 of the 16 breast tumors had positive estrogen receptors[4].

Nonetheless, all the studies must be analyzed with care to discover the existence of risk factors other than those resulting from the absence of pregnancy and lactation, which is common in the population of infertile patients[33–35].

Recently isolated cases of breast cancer after ovarian stimulation treatment have been published[36]. French national data of 24 cases of post-IVF breast cancer suggest a short interval between stimulation and the appearance of breast cancer, a low tumoral stage and good post-treatment development (18 patients in complete remission with a mean follow-up of 2.8 years)[37].

A different situation has been published by Arbour and colleagues[38]. They described a case of breast cancer which appeared 1 year after a post-IVF birth in a woman with a family history of family-based breast and ovarian cancer. The authors found that 92% of such cases are related to the presence of the *BRCA-1* gene.

OUR DATA

We have evaluated the incidence of gynecological cancer among the first 900 patients who underwent ovarian stimulation with a view to IVF in our Institute and who were followed up for more than 10 years (7917 years of follow-up). Among these patients we found two cases of breast cancer and one case of ovarian cancer. At the same time we analyzed the data of a historical group of five patients from our Service of Reproductive Medicine, who were not included above and who presented a gynecological cancer in their follow-up.

The first evaluation that we made was epidemiological, taking into account the expected incidence and that encountered in our sample with regard to the protection and risk factors presented by the patients included in the follow-up. We took as a standard or reference population the population of the province of Tarragona and obtained data from their cancer register during the period 1984–87. From these data we obtained an estimation of the expected cases, taking as a starting point the specific levels of incidence by age and sex from this register.

According to the data (Table 1) from our study population, 2.3 cases of breast cancer, 1.08 cases of ovarian cancer and 2.1 cases of endometrial cancer were expected. The observation of two breast cancer cases and one case of ovarian cancer does not give us standardized morbidity indices lower than unity, and we can therefore conclude that we have not observed more cases than would have been expected.

Influence of the patients' epidemiological data

We evaluated the histories of interest in the group of 897 patients who did not develop a gynecological cancer and compared them with those of the group of eight patients with

Table 1 Assisted reproduction techniques and later cancer. A total of 900 patients were studied and the total follow-up period was 7917 years

Type of cancer	*No. of observed cases*	*No. of expected cases*	*Standardized morbidity index*	*95% confidence interval*
Breast	2	2.30	0.86	0.3–2.1
Ovarian	1	1.08	0.92	0.9–2.7
Endometrial	—	2.10	—	—
Total	3	5.48	0.96	0.4–6.4

cancer (three included in the follow-up and five historical patients). As can be seen in Table 2, there were no differences between the two populations, except for a greater incidence of a first-grade family history of gynaecological cancer in the group of eight patients who developed a cancer (12.5%) than in the 897 patients who did not present with this condition (0.4%) ($p < 0.04$). The age at the end of the follow-up was greater in the group of patients with cancer (39.2 ± 4 years) than in the patients without the disease (36.3 ± 6 years) ($p < 0.008$).

Follow-up of patients

The incidence of post-treatment pregnancy was somewhat higher, though without reaching a level of statistical significance, in the group of patients without cancer (161/897; 17.9%) than in the patients who did develop the condition (1/8; 12.5%). The mean number of ovarian stimulation cycles was higher in the cancer group (3.1 ± 1.3) than in the group of healthy patients (1.5 ± 0.8) ($p < 0.0001$). Likewise, as shown in Table 3, the mean follow-up period until the appearance of the cancer or

Table 2 Epidemiological data

Risk factors	*Patients without a gynecological cancer* (%) ($n = 897$)	*Patients with a gynecological cancer* (%) ($n = 8$)
Previous family history of cancer	0.4	12.5*
Previous personal history	2.8	8.5
Previous pregnancies	6	—
Previous miscarriages	3.6	12.5

*$p < 0.04$

Table 3 Follow-up data. Values are given as mean ± SD, where appropriate

	Patients without a gynecological cancer ($n = 897$)	*Patients with a gynecological cancer* ($n = 8$)
Post-treatment pregnancy (n)	161 (17.9%)	1 (12.5%)
Final age (years)	36.3 ± 6	39.2 ± 4*
Treatment cycles (n)	1.5 ± 0.8	3.1 ± 1.3**
Follow-up period (years)	8.8 ± 2.3	4.5 ± 3.1***

*$p < 0.008$; **$p < 0.0001$; ***$p < 0.0007$

until the cessation of treatment was shorter in the group of patients with cancer (4.5 ± 3.1 years versus 8.8 ± 2.3 years) ($p < 0.0007$).

CONCLUSIONS

Great care must be taken in interpreting all these data, since some of the differences observed between the groups may be due to what are still very preliminary results, which may be affected by some statistical anomaly. For this reason, this study remains open to include more patients and extend their follow-up. Continued study of a large number of cases may change some of the trends or confirm others.

We must not forget the risk factors that these patients are subjected to by virtue of being infertile. In our study we have not been able to discern differences with respect to the incidence of post-treatment pregnancy between the two groups. We shall probably reach the conviction that much wider multicenter studies will be needed in order to draw definitive conclusions[39,40].

Nulliparity itself implies an increased risk of gynecological malignancies. If this condition is related to infertility, the risk increases even more. Nevertheless, infertile patients do not have an additional risk if they have undergone several cycles of ovarian stimulation protocols. Maybe there is a link between infertility and ovarian cancer related to ovarian functional abnormalities.

The lack of protection factors, such as pregnancy and lactation, will also increase the risk of the infertile population for other gynecological cancers. However, if these patients achieve a pregnancy after ART procedures, their risk will be low and comparable to that of fertile women[41].

REFERENCES

1. Lunenfeld B, Ron E. Cancer incidence in infertile women. *Hum Reprod* 1994;9(Suppl 4): 94
2. Shoham Z. Epidemiology, etiology and fertility drugs in ovarian epithelial carcinoma. Where are we today? *Fertil Steril* 1994;62:433–48
3. Schenker JG, Ezra Y. Complications of assisted reproductive techniques. *Fertil Steril* 1994; 61:411–22
4. Brzezinski A, Peretz T, Mor-Yosef J, Schenker J. Ovarian stimulation and breast cancer. Is there a link? *Gynecol Oncol* 1993;15:1–4
5. Ron E, Lunenfield B, Menczer J, *et al*. Blumstein T, Cancer incidence in a cohort of infertile women. *Am J Epidemiol* 1987;125:780–90

6. Lopes P, Julou V, Mensier A, *et al.* Cancer de l'ovaire et procreation médicalement assistée. *Contracept Fertil Sex* 1992;20:797–8
7. Whittemore AS, Wu ML, Paffenbarger RS, *et al.* Epithelial ovarian cancer and the ability to conceive. *Cancer Res* 1989;49:4047–52
8. Whittemore AS, Harris R, Itnyre J and the Collaborative Ovarian Cancer Group. Characteristics relating to ovarian cancer risk: collaborative analysis of 12 vs case–control studies. II. Invasive epithelial ovarian cancers in white women. *Am J Epidemiol* 1992;136: 1184–203
9. Whittemore AS, Harris R, Itnyre J, Halpern J and the Collaborative Ovarian Cancer Group. Characteristics relating to ovarian cancer risk: collaborative analysis of 12 vs case–control studies. I. Methods. *Am J Epidemiol* 1992;136:1175–83
10. Amso NN. Potential health hazards of assisted reproduction. Problems facing the clinician. *Hum Reprod* 1995;10:1628–30
11. Dargent D. Cancer de l'ovaire. Actualités. *Contracept Fertil Sex* 1995;23:122–6
12. Weiss NS, Lyon JL, Liff JM, Vollmer WM, Daling JR. Incidence of ovarian cancer in relation to the use of oral contraceptives. *Int J Cancer* 1981;28:669–71
13. Cramer DW, Hutchinson GB, Welch WR, Scully RE, Knaap RC. Factors affecting the association of oral contraceptives and ovarian cancer. *N Engl J Med* 1982;307:1047–51
14. Fathalla MF. Incessant ovulation: a factor in ovarian neoplasm. *Lancet* 1971;2:163
15. Negri E, Franceschi S, Tzonov A, Booth M, La Vecchia C, Trichopoulos D. Pooled analysis of 3 European case–control studies of ovarian factors. I. Reproductive factors and risk of epithelial ovarian cancer. *Int J Cancer* 1991;49:50–6
16. Whittemore AS. Fertility drugs and risk of ovarian cancer. *Hum Reprod* 1993;8:999–1000
17. Food and Drug Administration. FDA asks for fertility drug labelling change. FDA talk paper, 13 January 1993
18. Marrs RP, Hartz SC. Comments on the possible association between ovulation inducing agents and ovarian cancer. The *American Fertility Society*, Birmingham, Alabama, January 1993
19. Cohen J, Forman R, Harlap S, *et al.* IFFS Expert Group Report on the Whittemore study related to the risk of ovarian cancer associated with the use of infertility agents. *Hum Reprod* 1993;8:996–8
20. National Cancer Institute. *Cancer Facts. Fertility Drugs as a Risk Factor for Ovarian Cancer.* Bethesda, MD: National Institute of Child Health and Human Development, 13 January 1993
21. Stanford News Bureau. Ovarian cancer risk assessed in comprehensive study. *News Bureau.* Stanford, California: Stanford University Medical Center, 1 December 1993
22. Balasch J, Barri PN. Follicular stimulation and ovarian cancer? *Hum Reprod* 1993;8:990–6
23. Daya S. Risque de cancer de l'ovaire chez les femmes traitées pour infertilité. *Contracept Fertil Sex* 1994;22:593–6
24. Cruickshank DJ. Aetiological importance of ovulation in epithelial ovarian cancer: a population based study. *Br Med J* 1990;301:525–35
25. Balasch J, Peñarrubia J, Marquez M, *et al.* Ovulation side and ovarian cancer. *Gynecol Endocrinol* 1994;8:51–4

26. Rossing MA, Daling JR, Weiss NS, Moore DE, Self SC. Ovarian tumors in a cohort of infertile women. *N Engl J Med* 1994;331:771–6
27. Grimbizis G, Tarlatzis B, Bontis J, *et al.* Two cases of ovarian tumours in women who had undergone multiple ovarian stimulation attempts. *Hum Reprod* 1995;10:520–3
28. Mosgaard B, Lidegaard O, Kruger S, Schou G, Andersen A. Ovarian stimulation and borderline ovarian tumours: a case–control study. *Fertil Steril* 1998;70:1049–55
29. Duska L, Chang Y, Flynn CE, *et al.* Epthelial ovarian carcinoma in the reproductive age groups. *Cancer* 1999;85:2623–9
30. Mantzavinos T, Kanakas N, Genatas C, Papadias K, Zourlas P. Five years follow-up in two patients with borderline tumours of the ovary hyperstimulated by gonadotrophin therapy for *in vitro* fertilization. *Hum Reprod* 1994;9:2032–3
31. Franceschi S, Vecchia C, Negri E, *et al.* Fertility drugs and risk of epithelial ovarian cancer in Italy. *Hum Reprod* 1994;9:1673–5
32. Ron E, Boice JD Jr, Hamburger S, Stovall M. Mortality following radiation treatment for infertility of hormonal origin amenorrhea. *Int J Epidemiol* 1994;23:1165–73
33. Fernandez-Cid A, Dexeus S. Factores de riesgo elevado en patología mamaria. *Toko-Ginecol Pract* 1978;418:239–48
34. Fernandez-Cid A, Sentis J, Porteiro E, Petracco A, Gonzalez R. Edad y cáncer de mama. *Acta Ginecol* 1979;35:315–21
35. Fernandez-Cid A, Sentis J, Porteiro E, Petracco A. Factores de riesgo en patología mamaria. Estudio estadístico. *Acta Ginecol* 1980;36:89–110
36. Demetroulis C, Anastasiades K, Jayant G, Saridogan E. Fertility drugs for induction of ovulation and breast cancer. Is there a link? *Contracept Fertil Sex* 1995;23(Suppl 9):Special 1
37. Jourdain O, Avril A, Maurial L, Roux D, Commenges-Ducos M, Dallay D. Cancer du sein et traitement par HMG. Y-a-t-il un lien? *J Obstet Gynecol* 1995;3:230–1
38. Arbour L, Narod S, Glendon G, *et al. In vitro* fertilization and family history of breast cancer. *Lancet* 1994;344:610–11
39. Venn A, Watson L, Lumley J, Giles G, King C, Healey D. Breast and ovarian cancer incidence after infertility and IVF. *Lancet* 1995;346:995–1000
40. Potashnik G, Lerner-Geva L, Genkin L, Chetrit A, Lunenfeld E, Porath A. Fertility drugs and the risk of breast and ovarian cancers: results of a long-term follow-up study. *Fertil Steril* 1999;71:853–9
41. Balasch J. Estimulación folicular ovárica y riesgo de cáncer ginecológico. 1999; in press

11

Clinical implications of genetic counselling for inherited susceptibility to breast and ovarian cancer

S. Greggi, M. P. Paratore and M. Genuardi

INTRODUCTION

Genetic counselling is a multistep process through which both genetic and clinical information relative to a specific condition is conveyed to an individual. For adult-onset diseases, such as breast and ovarian cancer, genetic information consists of providing lifetime risk estimates of disease development in healthy family members. Such estimates are now often based on the results of genetic tests. Since these enable individuals who are susceptible to a specific disease to be identified, they have also been described as predictive tests. However, it must be stressed that the results of such tests are associated with considerable uncertainties, related to genetic and phenotypic heterogeneity, incomplete penetrance, variable age of onset, and the efficacy of preventive and surveillance options. Consequently, the entire process of information and counselling inevitably has a psychosocial impact on both the individual and his/her family, and may have lifetime negative behavioral effects.

EVALUATION OF FAMILIES FOR INHERITED BREAST AND OVARIAN CANCER RISK

Selected parameters must be considered in order to discriminate between high- and moderate-risk individuals/families. The following general characteristics are suggestive of an autosomal dominant predisposition:

(1) Presence of multiple breast and/or ovarian cancer cases in the pedigree;

(2) Early age at cancer diagnosis;

(3) Presence of multiple breast or breast plus ovarian tumors in the same individual.

The majority of subjects referred to a cancer genetics clinic belong to a moderate-risk category, not showing a striking family history. However, a subset of these may still have a genetic predisposition, which can be masked by a small family size, a low penetrance of specific mutations or by yet unspecified genetic or environmental modifying factors. Furthermore, some early-onset sporadic breast cancers may be caused by *de novo* germline mutations.

At this point, it is possible to provide risk estimates based either on Mendelian segregation (for high-risk individuals) or on risk prediction models (for moderate-risk individuals)[1] and to consider the opportunity of performing a genetic test. *BRCA1* and *BRCA2* are involved in most families with breast/ovarian cancer[2,3]. *BRCA1* mutations have been estimated to account for 88% of families with multiple cases of both breast and ovarian cancer[4]. On the other hand, *BRCA2* is specifically associated with male breast cancer occurrences[3]. The contribution of *BRCA1* and *BRCA2* to site-specific hereditary female breast cancer may be similar, each accounting for about one-third of the families, but results from linkage and mutation analyses indicate that other gene(s) are likely to be involved[5,6]. Rare familial aggregates of breast cancer are related to mutations in the *P53* or *PTEN* genes, which are associated with Li–Fraumeni and Cowden syndrome, respectively.

The frequency of *BRCA1* and *BRCA2* mutation carriers in the general population is low, ranging from 1/345[7] to 1/833[8] for *BRCA1*, and probably being much lower for *BRCA2*. These figures have been derived from population-based studies and await further confirmation from direct molecular investigations, which so far have been performed on selected patient groups. These preliminary investigations have shown that about 7.5% of breast cancer cases diagnosed before the age 35 years[9] and about 5% of ovarian cancer cases (< 70 years)[10] arise in carriers of *BRCA1* mutations.

Age-specific cumulative risks have been estimated for breast and ovarian cancer based on data from linkage studies and, more recently, from population-based case–control studies (Table 1). In addition, these mutations may confer slightly increased risks of other cancers, such as colon and prostate cancer in *BRCA1* mutation carriers[11] and pancreatic cancer in *BRCA2* mutation carriers[12].

Table 1 Risks of breast and ovarian cancer associated with *BRCA1* and *BRCA2* mutations

		Risk estimate (by the age of 70 years)	
Type of cancer	*Gene*	*Derived from high-risk families*	*Derived from population-based studies*
Breast (in women)	BRCA1	85%[11]	69%[7]
	BRCA2	85%[11]	—
Ovarian	BRCA1	44%* (36.3)	21%[7]
	BRCA2	< 10%[8]	—

*This is an average value. Ovarian cancer risk may depend on the type of *BRCA1* mutation

Finally, given the multifactorial etiology of cancer, other, non-genetic, factors may affect the individual risk. For instance, results from the Nurses' Health Study suggest that reproductive history may exert opposite effects on breast cancer risk in women with a positive family history relative to those without breast cancer cases in their families[13].

GENETIC TESTING

Based on the combination of these factors, it is possible to identify subjects eligible for *BRCA1/BRCA2* genetic testing (Table 2)[14], which is not currently carried out in the general population. Direct analysis of the *BRCA1* and *BRCA2* genes can allow the identification of pathogenetic mutations in at-risk individuals. However, currently available techniques are expensive and time-consuming, and their sensitivity levels are not defined. In fact, a negative test does not necessarily imply the absence of mutations, since these may be located in yet unexplored regions of the tested genes or in other, yet unknown, predisposing genes. Furthermore, a negative test result still leaves the individual exposed to the general population risk of developing breast or ovarian cancer.

On the other hand, the finding of a pathogenetic mutation does not provide definite answers to the individual's concerns. The presence of a mutation does not allow the prediction to be made of whether or when cancer will occur, nor does it lead to a uniform clinical approach for cancer risk reduction and early diagnosis (see below).

The only instance in which the result of genetic testing is clear-cut relates to a negative finding in an at-risk relative of a patient with an ascertained pathogenetic mutation. In this case, the individual is advised to adhere to the prevention and early diagnosis guidelines applicable to the general population.

PREVENTIVE OPTIONS AND CLINICAL SURVEILLANCE

Recently, the Cancer Genetics Studies Consortium, organized by the National Human Genome Research Institute, provided recommendations for cancer surveillance and risk reduction in *BRCA1* and *BRCA2* mutation carriers[15]. Several opportunities can be offered, none of which has proved to be efficient in follow-up care (Table 3).

Table 2 Eligibility for genetic testing. Prior probability of a *BRCA1* mutation estimated to be > 10%. From reference 14

Family with at least two breast cancer cases and one or more cases of ovarian cancer diagnosed at any age
Family with at least three breast cancers diagnosed before the age of 50 years
Sister pairs with two of the following cancers diagnosed before the age of 50 years: two breast cancers; two ovarian cancers; or a breast and an ovarian cancer
Relatives of individuals with breast cancer diagnosed before the age of 30 years

Table 3 Options for cancer prevention in *BRCA1–2* mutation carriers. From reference 15

Options	*Interval*	*Age at which option is offered*
Breast self-examination	monthly	≥ 18 years
Clinician breast examination	annually or 6-monthly	≥ 25 years
Mammography	annually	≥ 25 years
Pelvic examination	every 6 months	≥ 25–35 years
TV-USS with color Doppler and CA 125	every 6 months	≥ 25–35 years
Prostate cancer surveillance: rectal examination and PSA	annually	≥ 50 years
Flexibile sigmoidoscopy (or colonoscopy)	every 3–5 years	≥ 50 years
Prophylactic bilateral simple mastectomy (± reconstruction)	discussed as an option	
Prophylactic bilateral salpingo-oophorectomy	discussed as an option	

TV-USS, transvaginal ultrasound scan; PSA, prostate-specific antigen

Although a substantial reduction of breast cancer mortality has been proved following mammography screening, some considerations should be made with respect to the use of annual mammography in such a population subset. Data are controversial concerning an increased risk of cancer potentially associated with regular radiation exposure at an early age. However, the high risk of breast cancer harbored by *BRCA1–2* mutation carriers increases the likelihood that mammography is beneficial in these subjects, and it is suggested that the procedure is carried out annually beginning at the age of 30–35 years. Until now, the potential benefits of these measures are only based on expert opinion. However, because of the higher risk, members of families with breast/ovarian cancer family syndromes (with or without an ascertained germline mutation) are an ideal cohort for evaluating screening modalities.

Prophylactic surgery is another option to be discussed. There is no evidence to recommend for or against prophylactic bilateral simple mastectomy (PBSM) and/or oophorectomy (PBSO) as a measure for reducing breast/ovarian cancer risk. First, it should be pointed out that the risk of cancer development is not completely eliminated after organ removal. Failures have been reported following both these prophylactic procedures. In particular, breast cancer after PBSM (with or without reconstruction and nipple-sparing procedures) ranges from 1% to approximately 20% and it probably depends on the amount of residual (post-mastectomy) breast tissue[16,17]. Morever, it has to be considered that in most series the breast cancer risk category (e.g. family history, mutational status) and the surgical procedure adopted are undetermined, and the follow-up duration is very variable[16,17].

Both the US National Institutes of Health[18] and the American College of Obstetricians and Gynecologists[19] have recommended PBSO in *BRCA1* mutation carriers and in women with a documented family history suggesting a site-specific ovarian, a breast/ovarian or a Lynch II syndrome. Bilateral oophorectomy is also an option for *BRCA2* mutation carriers, but their lower risk reduces the likelihood of benefit[15]. After the observation of intra-abdominal carcinomatosis following PBSO[20], the effectiveness of the procedure has been analyzed in different studies. Failure rates ranging from 2% to 11%[21] have recently been reported. The observed-to-expected ratio was 13 : 1 (1–47) compared to 24 : 1 (10–47) in a control group not submitted to PBSO[22]. The optimal age for such procedures has not yet been established. However, PBSM and PBSO procedures are generally offered after the age of 40 years (or less in the case of breast/ovarian cancer at a younger age in first-degree relatives) or after completion of childbearing.

No data are available on the effects of estrogen/progestagen therapy on the ovarian and breast cancer risk in *BRCA1–2* mutation carriers. Several studies on oral contraceptives demonstrated a 40–50% ovarian cancer risk reduction, depending on the duration of use (5–9 years; > 10 years), including women with a family history of ovarian cancer[23]. On the other hand, a slight increase in breast cancer risk has been observed in oral contraceptive users, but with no long-term effects[24].

Again, there are no recommendations available concerning the use or avoidance of estrogen replacement therapy by *BRCA1–2* mutation carriers and members of families with breast/ovarian cancer syndrome, regardless of an ascertained germline mutation. It has been reported that long-term (≥ 7–10 years) use of estrogen replacement therapy is associated with a significant increase of breast cancer risk (relative risk 1.3)[25]. Moreover, an increased life expectancy has been estimated in the general population – but not in breast cancer high-risk subjects – when estrogen-related benefits (e.g. decreased risks of osteoporosis and cardiopathy) are taken into account[26]. The concerns above are particularly important when long-term estrogen replacement therapy is being considered in women undergoing PBSO at an early age.

As to cancers of other sites, the increase in risk is probably not sufficiently high to justify strict monitoring. Carriers of *BRCA1* mutations should be informed about the slightly increased risk of prostate and colon cancer, and encouraged to adhere to the recommendations issued for the general population, which are quite controversial for prostate carcinoma. Currently, there are no data available on pancreatic cancer risk in *BRCA2* mutation carriers, but, because of its relatively low entity and the absence of means for adequate early diagnosis, there are no recommendations about monitoring of any type.

COUNSELLING APPROACHES

The approach is multidisciplinary and involves the participation of several professional personnel, including medical geneticists, genetic counsellors, clinicians and psychologists.

Because of the widespread use of molecular tests for several disorders, it is now possible to ascertain whether an individual is genetically susceptible to a specific disease. However, genetic testing and counselling are not carried out exactly in parallel – the latter begins before and continues after the former has been performed. The clinical, social and psychological implications of genetic testing have to be addressed beforehand, and follow-up after testing is also an essential component of counselling.

The entire process can thus be subdivided into three steps:

(1) Pre-test counselling;

(2) Genetic testing, including disclosure of the results;

(3) Post-test follow-up.

The pre-test phase should start well before (weeks or months) genetic testing. At this time, the individual receives basic information on the transmission of genetic diseases, as well as details on the specific condition for which counselling is required, including information on early diagnosis, prevention and available treatments. At the same time, the procedure of genetic testing is described, along with the significance of any potential result, positive or negative, including sensitivity and specificity limits. The potential consequences of the result on insurance coverage and job opportunities need to be discussed at this moment, since these may play an important role in further decisions. Another issue to be addressed is that of the potential psychological effects of testing on the individual and on family relationships. Testing for breast and ovarian cancer is associated with peculiar psychological aspects, which are also partly related to the preventive surgical options included among the possible alternatives for risk reduction. Brochures resuming all topics discussed at the time of the first meeting should be provided to the patient being counselled. At least one more pre-test meeting is usually scheduled, during which the counsellor verifies that the information has been appropriately received. At this point, the decision on whether or not to undergo testing can be taken by the patient, who should be aware that she can change her mind about receiving the results at any time. Once the blood sample has been drawn, the patient should be contacted again to make sure that she still wants to have the results disclosed.

Reactions to the results are strongly influenced by their outcome. A negative test usually has beneficial and reassuring effects, with a decrease in depressive symptoms[27], although in some instances it may cause the appearance of guilt feelings for not being a carrier while other relatives have already developed the disease or have been provided with a positive result. The reaction to a positive result is less predictable, but it has been observed that most subjects do not show an increase in depression[27]. This outcome is not completely unexpected, since during pre-test sessions it has emerged that one of the most common reasons to undergo genetic testing is an expectation of relief from uncertainty about the risk[28].

At the after-test follow-up, one should again verify that the information on the test result has been correctly perceived, and, where the test is positive, all necessary assistance should be given to make the appropriate choice about the preventive and early diagnosis options and to cope with the psychosocial consequences. Genetic counselling for susceptibility to breast and ovarian cancer in the molecular genetics era is still in its infancy.

Preliminary data from counselling studies indicate great expectations from the public. Nevertheless, it has recently been reported that only 43% of women belonging to hereditary breast/ovarian cancer families requested results of *BRCA1–2* testing[27]. This is probably due to the limitations of the genetic test, and to the lack of easy, harmless and effective means of cancer prevention and screening. Rigorous co-operative studies are needed over several years to adequately assess the cost-effectiveness of genetic testing. Moreover, in Italy, as in all other European countries, no funds are available from National Health Services for such an analysis, and the likelihood that research laboratories will be able to undertake a study of this kind on a large scale seems to be very poor. On the other hand, results of prospective studies, once available, will be useful for offering high-risk individuals more precise strategies for cancer prevention.

REFERENCES

1. Claus EB, Risch N, Thompson WD. Autosomal dominant inheritance of early onset breast cancer. *Cancer* 1994;73:643–51
2. Easton DF, Bishop DT, Ford D, Crockford DP, and the Breast Cancer Linkage Consortium. Genetic linkage analysis in familial breast and ovarian cancer: results from 214 families. *Am J Hum Genet* 1993;52:678–701
3. Wooster R, Neuhausen SL, Mangion J, *et al.* Localization of a breast cancer susceptibility gene, *BRCA2*, to chromosome 13q12–13. *Science* 1994;265:2088–90
4. Narod SA, Ford D, Devilee P, *et al.* An evaluation of genetic heterogeneity in 145 breast–ovarian cancer families. *Am J Hum Genet* 1995;56:254–64
5. Marcus JN, Watson P, Page DL, *et al.* Hereditary breast cancer. Pathology, prognosis and *BRCA1* and *BRCA2* gene linkage. *Cancer* 1996;77:697
6. Serova OM, Mazoyer S, Puget N, *et al.* Mutations in *BRCA1* and *BRCA2* in breast cancer families: are there more breast cancer-susceptibility genes? *Am J Hum Genet* 1997;60: 486–95
7. Whittemore A, Gong G, Itnyre J. Prevalence and contribution of *BRCA1* mutations in breast cancer and ovarian cancer: results from three US population-based case–control studies of ovarian cancer. *Am J Hum Genet* 1997;60:496–504
8. Ford D, Easton DF, Peto J. Estimates of the gene frequency of *BRCA1* and its contribution to breast and ovarian cancer incidence. *Am J Hum Genet* 1995;57:1457
9. Langston AA, Malone KE, Thompson JD, *et al.* *BRCA1* mutations in a population-based sample of young women with breast cancer. *N Engl J Med* 1996;334:137
10. Stratton JF, Gayther SA, Russell P, *et al.* Contribution of *BRCA1* mutations to ovarian cancer. *N Engl J Med* 1997;336:1125–30

11. Ford D, Easton DF, Bishop DT, *et al.*, and the Breast Cancer Linkage Consortium. Risk of Cancer in *BRCA1*-mutation carriers. *Lancet* 1994;343:692–5
12. Thorlacius S, Olafsdottir G, Tryggvadottir L, *et al.* A single *BRCA2* mutation in male and female breast cancer families from Iceland with varied cancer phenotypes. *Nature Genet* 1996;13:117
13. Colditz GA, Rosner BA, Speizer FE. Risk factors for breast cancer according to family history of breast cancer. *J Natl Cancer Inst* 1996;88:365–71
14. Commentary on the American Society of Clinical Oncology Statement on Genetic Testing for Cancer Susceptibility. *J Clin Oncol* 1996;14:1737–40
15. Burke W, Daly M, Garber J, *et al.* Recommendations for follow-up care of individuals with an inherited predisposition to cancer. *J Am Med Assoc* 1997;277:997–1003
16. Bilimoria MM, Morrow M. The woman at increased risk for breast cancer: evaluation and management strategies. *CA Cancer J Clin* 1995;45:263–78
17. Humphrey LJ. Subcutaneous mastectomy is not a prophylaxis against carcinoma of the breast: opinion or knowledge? *Am J Surg* 1983;145:311–12
18. National Institutes of Health Consensus Development Panel on Ovarian Cancer. Ovarian cancer: screening, treatment, and follow-up. *J Am Med Assoc* 1995;273:491–7
19. American College of Obstetricians and Gynecologists. *Int J Gynecol Obstet* 1996;52:101–2
20. Tobacman JK, Tucker MA, Kase R. Intraabdominal carcinomatosis after prophylactic oophorectomy in ovarian cancer prone families. *Lancet* 1982;2:795–7
21. Piver MS, Jishi MF, Tsukada Y, *et al.* Primary peritoneal carcinoma after prophylactic oophorectomy in women with a family history of ovarian cancer. *Cancer* 1993;71:2651–5
22. Struewing JP, Watson P, Easton DF. Prophylactic oophorectomy in inherited breast/ovarian cancer families. *J Natl Cancer Inst Monogr* 1995;17:33–5
23. Gross TO, Schlesselman JJ. The estimated effect of oral contraceptive use on the cumulative risk of epithelial ovarian cancer. *Obstet Gynecol* 1994;83:419–24
24. Collaborative Group on Hormonal Factors in Breast Cancer. Breast cancer and hormonal contraceptives. *Lancet* 1996;347:1713–27
25. Grady D, Rubin S, Petitti DB, *et al.* Hormone therapy to prevent disease and prolong life in post-menopausal women. *Ann Intern Med* 1992;117:1016–37
26. Division of Cancer Prevention and Control. *Clinical Trials of Hormone Replacement Therapy in Patients with a History of Breast Cancer.* Minutes of a working group. Bethesda, MD: National Cancer Institute, 1993
27. Lerman C, Narod S, Schulman K, *et al.* *BRCA1* testing in families with hereditary breast–ovarian cancer. A prospective study of patient decision making and outcomes. *J Am Med Assoc* 1996;275:1885–92
28. Lerman C, Biesecker B, Benkendorf JL, *et al.* Controlled trial of pretest education approaches to enhance informed decision-making for *BRCA1* gene testing. *J Natl Cancer Inst* 1997;89:148–57

12

BRCA1/2 mutation carriers and women at high risk for breast and ovarian cancer: preventive and therapeutic implications

M. W. Beckmann, B. Kuschel and H. G. Bender

INTRODUCTION

Breast cancer is the major cancer disease for women in Western countries and the leading cause of death in women between the ages 40 and 55 years[1]. Women with a family history of breast cancer – especially at a young age, with bilateral disease or with multiple affected family members – are at increased risk for breast cancer. Hereditary breast cancer is estimated to represent approximately 5–15% of diagnosed breast cancer cases. In contrast, ovarian cancer is a rare disease – about one in 80 women will be diagnosed during their lifetime. Overall, hereditary ovarian cancer is an uncommon disease, but women with first-degree relatives affected by ovarian cancer and/or breast cancer are at increased risk of getting ovarian cancer. Germline mutations of *TP53* (Li–Fraumeni syndrome), *ATM* (ataxia–telangiectasia-mutated gene) and *PTEN* (Cowden syndrome) are found in the minority, whilst germline mutations of the susceptibility genes *BRCA1* and *BRCA2* are found in the majority of the familial breast and ovarian cancer syndrome cases[2]. According to synopsis studies of the Breast Cancer Linkage Consortium (BCLC), breast cancer lifetime risk for *BRCA1* mutation carriers by the age of 70 years is 82% (general population risk 8–10%), and for *BRCA2* mutation carriers it is 84% in high-penetrant cancer families. Ovarian cancer lifetime risk for *BRCA1* mutation carriers by age 70 years is 44%, and for *BRCA2* mutation carriers it is 17%[3,4]. In mutation carriers, lifetime risk may vary due to modifying genes, environmental factors and allelic heterogeneity.

Members from high-risk families are frightened about breast and/or ovarian cancer by personal and familial experiences. Therefore, participation in chemopreventive trials or preventive measures such as prophylactic bilateral mastectomy and/or prophylactic bilateral salpingo-oophorectomy are serious considerations and potential options discussed by the women at risk either with the physician-in-charge, the oncospecialist or a member of a cancer genetics clinic. Data from prospective randomized trials evaluating medical prevention in cancer-prone individuals, as well as the effects and consequences of prophylactic bilateral mastectomy and/or prophylactic bilateral salpingo-oophorectomy, are not yet available.

Arguments for and against preventive and therapeutic options are based on clinical experiences, lifetime data from women with sporadic breast cancer and/or ovarian cancer, and on theoretical tumor biological findings.

Individual considerations for the choice of options include:

(1) Individual risk assessment and gain in life expectancy;

(2) Screening and early cancer detection methods;

(3) Medical prevention;

(4) Disease characteristics and prognosis;

(5) Surgical prevention;

(6) Anxiety and quality of life.

INDIVIDUAL RISK ASSESSMENT AND GAIN IN LIFE EXPECTANCY

For women with multiple family members affected by breast cancer, ovarian cancer or other cancer types, questions arise about their individual breast cancer and/or ovarian cancer risk and the time of disease onset. Risk assessment starts with an estimation of probabilities based on the breast cancer/ovarian cancer diagnosis, the type of inheritance, information about the family history, linkage results from genetic marker studies and the results from genetic testing, including information about test sensitivity and specificity. All risk estimates extrapolate risk data from defined and, at best, mutation-tested cohorts for both mutation carrier probability and overall disease risk[3–6]. Various risk-assessment models are applied for breast cancer, including the Gail model, the Claus model and the Bayes' theorem, most of which are based on different prerequisite assumptions[7–9]. However, most of these models are not able to take into account individual modulating anamnestic breast cancer risk factors, i.e. early menarche, late age at first childbirth, late menopause, history of benign breast disease and lifestyle, including nutrition, alcohol or smoking, or consider the heterogeneity of the disease. For ovarian cancer risk assessment, no statistical model is available. Therefore, statistical and anamnestic risk assessment remains inaccurate and difficult to interpret. Whether calculated differences of a 40%, 60% or 70% *a priori* risk are of importance for the individual woman, or whether the calculated differences in risk assessment will influence her decision whether or not to take preventive or prophylactic measures, is unclear.

The gain in life expectancy is a measure of the effectiveness of medical interventions, but its interpretation requires that it be placed in the population context[10]. The interpretation of life expectancy gain is particulary problematic for preventive interventions, for which the gain is often just weeks or even days when averaged across the entire target population. Life-saving effectiveness compares the full survival curves of a treatment and a control group. The gain in life expectancy as a measure of outcome is the shift in the survival curve caused by the intervention. Mathematically, the gain in life expectancy is the area between the curves of both group. This area is measured in two dimensions, compared to the usual one-dimension evaluations: the gain in median survival time (horizontal gain) or the gain in survival probability at 5 years (vertical gain). Comparing different intervention strategies, a gain in life expectancy of 1 month from a preventive intervention targeted at a population at average risk, and a gain of 1 year in a population at elevated risk, can both be considered large[10]. For example, in populations at average risk, 10 years of biennial mammography for a 50-year-old woman gives a gain in life expectancy of 0.8 months. In contrast, in a population at high risk for a hip fracture, combined hormone replacement therapy (HRT) for a 50-year-old woman gives a gain in life expectancy of 2–13 months. Similarly, a biopsy to evaluate postmenopausal bleeding followed by dilatation and curettage or hysterectomy for a 50-year-old woman gives a life expectancy gain of 6 months, while the same procedures for a 70-year-old woman give a gain in life expectancy of 2.2 months. When making a decision whether or not to undergo prophylactic bilateral mastectomy, the applied Markov process estimates the effect of an intervention based on a range of information about the incidence of breast cancer (i.e. modulation of risk according to different populations, including young Ashkenazi Jewish women), the prognosis of breast cancer and the efficacy of prophylactic surgery, including survival, quality of life and cost-effectiveness[11,12]. Young women (30 years) who test positive for the *BRCA1* and *BRCA2* gene mutations have a gain in life expectancy of 2.9–5.3 years[11] or 2.8–2.9 years[12], respectively. These gains vary with concomitant prophylactic bilateral salpingo-oophorectomy (3.2–7.6 years according to reference 11; 3.3–6.0 years

Table 1 Estimation of overall survival (years) and gain in life expectancy after prophylactic bilateral mastectomy (PBM)[11,12], compared to gain in life expectancy after chemotherapy (CHT) in breast cancer patients with and without lymph-node involvement (LN+/–)[10]

	Overall survival without PBM (years)	*Gain in life expectancy with PBM* (years)	*Gain in life expectancy with PBM and PBSO* (years)	*Gain in life expectancy with CHT* (years)	
				LN+	*LN–*
Schrag *et al.*[11]					
low-risk women	75.9	+ 2.9	+ 3.2		
high-risk women	67.5	+ 5.3	+ 7.6		
Grann *et al.*[12]					
low-risk women		+ 2.9	+ 3.3		
high-risk women		+ 2.8	+ 6.0		
Wright and Weinstein[10]				+ 0.3	+ 0.8

PBSO, prophylactic bilateral salpingo-oophorectomy

Table 2 Estimation of overall survival (years) and gain in life expectancy after prophylactic bilateral salpingo-oophorectomy (PBSO)[11,12], compared to gain in life expectancy after chemotherapy (CHT) in breast cancer patients with and without lymph-node involvement (LN+/–)[10]

	Overall survival without PBSO (years)	*Gain in life expectancy with PBSO* (years)	*Gain in life expectancy with PBSO and PBM* (years)	*Gain in life expectancy with CHT* (years)	
				LN+	*LN–*
Schrag *et al.*[11]					
low-risk women	75.9	+ 0.3	+ 3.2		
high-risk women	67.5	+ 1.7	+ 7.6		
Grann *et al.*[12]					
low-risk women		+ 0.4	+ 3.3		
high-risk women		+ 2.6	+ 6.0		
Wright and Weinstein[10]				+ 0.3	+ 0.8

PBM, prophylactic bilateral mastectomy

according to reference 12) (Tables 1 and 2). Unless the breast cancer risk is high, bilateral prophylactic surgery provides no significant benefit for the quality of life, but is cost-effective for the years of life saved compared with other medical interventions (e.g. medical prevention) that are deemed cost-effective[12].

SCREENING AND EARLY CANCER DETECTION METHODS

Despite high-quality randomized trials, the balance of harm and benefit attributable to breast cancer screening, including that in high-risk women, is yet unknown. Breast self-examination, breast examination by a clinician, mammography, breast ultrasound or magnetic resonance tomography (MRT) are potential screening methods for low- and high-risk populations[13–15]. The screening benefit of breast self-examination or breast examination by a clinician is not proven, even though more than 60% of all breast cancer cases are detected by the identification of a palpable breast mass. A meta-analysis of 13 randomized clinical trials using X-ray mamography showed that, in women between the ages of 50 and 74 years, the risk of dying from breast cancer is reduced by 26% (95% confidence interval (CI) 17–34%)[16,17]. There is also the risk of a false-positive X-ray mamography result in this age group[18], but this should not dissuade women above 50 years of age from undergoing X-ray mamography screening. In contrast, the benefit of X-ray mamography screening in women 40 to 49 years of age is still unclear. In randomized trials, the rate of death from breast cancer was the same in the screened group as in the control group for 7–10 years after the first X-ray mamography screening[16]. Thereafter (12–14 years after the first X-ray mamography screening), the women being postmenopausal at the time of screening, a reduction of mortality of 16% could be demonstrated. Therefore, X-ray mamography screening in the 40–49-year-old age group, or even in younger women at risk, is still under intense debate[14,19,20]. Increased breast density and cyclic hormonal variations are the major conflicting factors in this age group, decreasing X-ray mamography sensitivity and specificity[20–22]. Breast ultrasound or MRT may be potential diagnostic options for high-risk women, but, to date, their effect is only demonstrated in selective cohorts – prospective randomized trials are pending[20,23,24].

Standard recommendations for persons at risk for ovarian cancer include pelvic examination and transvaginal ultrasound imaging. Neither of these methods has proved to be effective as an ovarian cancer screening modality. Most ovarian cancer cases present at an advanced stage of disease, highlighting the need for effective early diagnostic tests. The serum marker CA 125 is under debate, with a slightly greater specifity in postmenopausal women[25]. Whereas pelvic examination is completely dependent on the examiner's skill, the transvaginal ultrasound technique is estimated to have a sensitivity of 80–90%. A review of ultrasound screening of over 13 000 asymptomatic women revealed that 17 ovarian cancer cases were detected, 15 with stage I disease. However, the major limitations of this screening approach were the false-positive results in 84 of 90 women with suspicious transvaginal ultrasound findings[26]. The option of starting ovarian cancer screening after the age of 35 years to avoid unnecessary biopsies may be challenged by findings from ovarian cancer patients from families with a strong ovarian cancer family history. They tend to develop ovarian cancer at a younger age than expected[27].

MEDICAL PREVENTION

Primary medical prevention ofbreast cancer aims at varying the endocrine, autocrine or paracrine environment of the breast tissue. Aromatase inhibitors, retinoids, isoflavonoids, or gonadotropin releasing hormone plus add-back low-dose oral contraceptives or HRT have been tested[23]. Published breast cancer prevention trials (National Surgical Adjuvant Breast and Bowel Project (NSABP) Breast Cancer Prevention Trial, BCPT-P1[28]; Royal Marsden Hospital Tamoxifen Randomised Chemoprevention Trial[29]; Italian Randomized Trial Among Hysterectomized Women[30]) tested tamoxifen 20 mg/day versus placebo according to specific breast cancer risk profiles. The BCPT-P1 trial demonstrated a significant reduction in breast cancer, but neither the Royal Marsden Hospital trial nor the Italian trial demonstrated this reduction in breast cancer (Table 3). Miscellaneous reasons for the interpretation of these data have to be considered, including differences in statistical variables (age, compliance, follow-up period and additional intake of HRT) and inclusion criteria or risk evaluation[23]. The BCPT-P1 trial used the Gail model for risk evaluation, the Royal Marsden trial used the family history (the strongest breast cancer risk factor of all), and the Italian trial used primarily the hysterectomy criteria and secondarily the family history. Subgroup

Table 3 Comparision between three published chemoprevention trials for breast cancer

	Studies		
	Fisher et al.[28] (n = 13 175)	*Powles et al.*[29] (n = 2471)	*Veronesi et al.*[30] (n = 3837)
Follow-up (woman years)	46 858	12 355	20 731
Median follow-up period (months)	48	70	46
Breast cancer cases			
total n	368	70	41
women with placebo (n)	244	36	22
women with tamoxifen treatment (n)	124	34	19
p value	0.00001	0.8	0.6358
Number of breast cancer cases/1000 woman years			
women with placebo (n)	6.6	5.0	2.3
women with tamoxifen treatment (n)	3.6	4.7	2.1

Table 4 Number of relatives with breast cancer (BC) in three published chemoprevention trials

	Studies		
	Fisher et al.[28]	*Powles et al.*[29]	*Veronesi et al.*[30]
Number of first-degree relatives < 50 years of age	—	1364 (55%)	—
Number of first-degree BC relatives			
0	3135 (24%)	100 (4%)	2713 (79%)
1	7485 (57%)	1845 (74%)	976 (18%)
2	2161 (16%)	374 (15%)	132 (3%)
≥ 3	394 (3%)	175 (7%)	16 (0.5%)

analysis for the evaluation of the effect of chemoprevention on women at high risk shows that the Royal Marsden trial included the most women with elevated risk according to the number of affected family members (Table 4). Family history as a risk factor can be neglected in the Italian trial. A total of 2503 (19%) women in the BCPT-P1 trial and 898 (36%) in the Royal Marsden trial have an 80% breast cancer risk according to the Claus model[31]. In this high-risk subgroup, 103 women (28% of all breast cancer cases) in the BCPT-P1 trial and 42 women (60% of all breast cancer cases) in the Royal Marsden trial developed breast cancer. Therefore, compared to the placebo group, the effect of chemoprevention can only be demonstrated in low- or medium-risk women, and not in the subgroup of women with high risk. According to the calculations of the above-described prevention trials, 6600 healthy women at low or medium risk must take tamoxifen to prevent 82 small, node-negative, estrogen receptor (ER)-positive breast cancer cases.

Based on the known protective effect of parity, the development of ovarian cancer is correlated to the rapid turnover and repair by epithelial cells after ovulation. The risk of ovarian cancer is reduced by 50% and the mortality by 80% in long-term users of oral contraceptive pills[32,33]. Therefore, oral contraceptive pills as a potential preventive measure for women at high risk of ovarian cancer may be an option. Indeed, a case–control study comparing 207 *BRCA1* or *BRCA2* mutation carriers with ovarian cancer to their 161 sisters showed a significant ovarian cancer risk reduction of 68% in oral contraceptive pill users after a period of 6 years or more[34]. Therefore, oral contraceptive pills may be considered as a part of cancer prevention programs for women with *BRCA1/2* mutations, but without prophylactic bilateral salpingo-oophorectomy. On the other hand, oral contraceptive pill use has an increasing effect on breast cancer incidence (relative risk (RR) in current users 1.24, 95% CI 1.15–1.23)[35]. Mortality during oral contraceptive pill use and in the first 10 years post-oral contraceptive pill use ceases (1–4 years after stopping: RR 1.16, 95% CI 1.08–1.23; 5–9 years after stopping: RR 1.07, 95% CI 1.02–1.13). For women who stopped use 10 or more years ago, no significant, either overall or for any specific cause of death, could be demonstrated[33]. The Collaborative Study on Hormonal Factors, which looked at 53 297 women with and 100 239 without breast cancer, demonstrated no variation of risk for women with or without a family history of breast cancer[35]. Data from small studies suggest, with marginal statistical significance, an increased breast cancer risk in the subset of mutation carriers or women with a breast cancer family history[36,37].

DISEASE CHARACTERISTICS AND PROGNOSIS

Clinical features of familial breast cancer patients defined by family history or mutation status show that the median age of breast cancer onset ranges from 40 to 50 years in *BRCA1* (42 ± 11 years) and *BRCA2* (47 ± 15 years) mutation carriers, whereas it is 60–70 years in patients with sporadic breast cancer (63 ± 14 years)[38,39]. *BRCA1* mutations are present in only approximately 10% of women with sporadic early-onset breast cancer (< 35 years). Bilateral (0.5% for sporadic versus 4.1–13% for *BRCA1/2* mutation carriers; $p < 0.001$) and contralateral (4–5.6% for sporadic versus 20–31% for *BRCA1/2* mutation carriers; $p < 0.01$) breast cancer is significantly more frequent among mutation carriers[39–42]. *BRCA1/2* mutation carriers may have higher rates of pregnancy-associated breast cancer (14 (21%) of 47 cases of breast cancer in *BRCA1/2* mutation carriers < 40 years of age versus 14 (6%) of 250 sporadic breast cancer cases < 40 years of age)[43].

Lobular *in situ*, medullary, tubular and lobular invasive carcinoma have been reported to be associated with a family history of breast cancer[44–46]. Breast cancer due to *BRCA1* mutations are significantly more often of the medullary subtype (up to 13% versus 2–4% in sporadic cases; $p < 0.01$) and with a prominent lymphocyte infiltration[39,47–49]. Ductal carcinoma *in situ* seems to be less associated with a family history of breast cancer (56% in sporadic versus 41% in *BRCA1* cases; $p = 0.001$)[47,48]. *BRCA1*-associated breast cancers are characterized by numerous mitoses, a pleomorphic pattern, higher proliferation rates, poor differentiation and histoprognostic grade 3[41–43,47,48,50], as well as a lack of ER (ER-negative breast cancers 64–90%; $p < 0.04$) and progesterone receptor (PR) (PR-negative breast cancers 70%; $p < 0.05$) expression[41–43,50] (Table 5). The significantly reduced PR and cyclin D_1 expression suggests an alteration of the transactivating function of ER in these tumors[51].

Molecular differences in *BRCA1/2*-associated tumors show specific somatic genetic changes in the 4q and 5q chromosomal regions in *BRCA1* tumors and in the 6q

Table 5 Differences in pathological tumor and steroid-hormone receptor characteristics between sporadic and hereditary breast cancer (BC) due to *BRCA1* and *BRCA2* mutations, based on different study data

	Sporadic BC		*BRCA1/BRCA2-associated BC*		
	Total n	*n (% cases)*	*Total n*	*n (% cases)*	*p Value*
Grading		*Grade 3*		*Grade 3*	
Ansquer *et al.*[41]	108	26 (24%)	15	11 (73%)	< 0.05
Robson *et al.*[42]	54	32 (59%)	21	21 (100%)	0.0002
Lakhani *et al.*[47]	368	133 (36%)	139/58	92 (66%)/24 (41%)	< 0.0001/0.04
ER expression		*ER-negative*		*ER-negative*	
Ansquer *et al.*[41]	108	40 (37%)	15	14 (93%)	< 0.04
Verhoog *et al.*[40]	150	52 (35%)	25	16 (64%)	0.005
Robson *et al.*[42]	56	19 (34%)	23	16 (70%)	0.006
PR expression		*PR-negative*		*PR-negative*	
Ansquer *et al.*[41]	108	38 (35%)	15	11 (73%)	< 0.05
Verhoog *et al.*[40]	133	45 (34%)	20	14 (70%)	0.002
Robson *et al.*[42]	55	26 (47%)	23	16 (70%)	0.09

ER, estrogen receptor; PR, progesterone receptor

and 13q regions in *BRCA2* tumors. In prophylactically removed breasts of high-risk women, cytogenetic abnormalities (loss of 3p12–14) and chromosomal aberrations (1q14, 3p14) have been detected[52,53]. These chromosomal regions may pinpoint genes in which inactivation (tumor-suppressor genes) or activation (oncogenes) promotes tumor progression in individuals predisposed to breast cancer[54,55]. *BRCA1*-associated breast tumors lack *Her-2/neu* expression, but show a high rate of *TP53* mutations[50].

Some studies looking at patients with a family history of breast cancer compared to women with sporadic cases of breast cancer have demonstrated no differences in disease-free survival. The prognosis of *BRCA1*-associated breast cancer compared to sporadic breast cancer cases is, as yet, unknown[39–42,44] (Table 6). This suggests a paradox: on the one hand, decreased disease-free survival and, on the other, increased overall survival in *BRCA1/2* mutation carriers, even though tumor characteristics predict aggressive tumor behavior and a poor prognosis (higher proliferation rates and a lack of steroid hormone receptors). High cellular fragility with a lack of DNA repair mechanisms may result in a better response to chemo- and radiotherapy. However, molecular findings may indicate a less likely response to endocrine therapeutic manipulation or chemopreventive agents such as tamoxifen, raloxifen and retinoids.

Table 6 Differences in survival between sporadic and hereditary breast cancer (BC) cases due to the *BRCA1/2* mutation status

	Sporadic BC		*BRCA1/BRCA2-associated BC*		
	Total n	*n (% cases)*	*Total n*	*n (% cases)*	*p Value*
Disease-free survival					
Verhoog *et al.*[40] (5 years of follow-up)	196	96 (49%)	49	25 (51%)	0.96
Robson *et al.*[42] (5 years of follow-up)	61	37 (31%)	30	11 (37%)	NS
Overall survival					
Marcus *et al.*[31] (3.6–8.3 years of follow-up)	130	61 (47%)	72/66	57 (79%)/42 (64%)	NS
Gaffney *et al.*[39] (5 years of follow-up)	50	35 (70%)	30/20	23 (77%)/15 (75%)	0.88
Verhoog *et al.*[40] (5 years of follow-up)	196	135 (69%)	49	31 (63%)	< 0.04
Ansquer *et al.*[41] (3.6 years of follow-up)	108	86 (80%)	15	9 (60%)	

NS, not significant

The risk for ovarian cancer is strongly associated with family history of the disease. Family members tend to develop their cancer at a younger age[27]. *BRCA1/2* mutation carriers with ovarian cancer or breast cancer/ovarian cancer ($n = 151$) tend to have a similar overall survival compared to families without an identified mutation ($n = 119$), whereas the survival in familial cases is estimated to be significantly worse than age-matched control cases without a family history of the disease. Histopathological findings revealed no differences in type, grade or stage according to the mutation status[56]. In comparison to sporadic ovarian cancer cases, familial ovarian cancer showed a mucinous type less frequently (2% versus 12%, $p < 0.001$) and presented more often with advanced disease[56] (Table 7). This, and the worse survival rates of familial ovarian cancer, may be a hint that familial ovarian cancer has a different biological structure and is more aggressive than sporadic ovarian cancer. Recent studies have reported the presence of premalignant lesions in ovaries prophylactically removed for familial cancer history[57,58]. However, no differences between prophylactically removed ovaries of *BRCA1/2* mutation carriers and women at familial risk could be identified[59].

Table 7 Survival differences between sporadic, familial and hereditary ovarian cancer (OC) due to the *BRCA1/2* mutation status

	Sporadic OC n (% of cases with 5-year survival)	*Familial OC n (% of cases with 5-year survival)*	*BRCA1-associated OC n (% of cases with 5-year survival)*	*BRCA2-associated OC n (% of cases with 5-year survival)*	*p Value*
Buller *et al.*[71]	34 (17%)	11 (67%)	ND (ND)	ND (ND)	< 0.04
Chang *et al.*[72]	84 (ND)	28 (ND)	ND (ND)	ND (ND)	NS
Rubin *et al.*[73]	ND (15%)	ND (ND)	53 (60%)	ND (ND)	< 0.001
Brunet *et al.*[74]	ND (ND)	ND (ND)	44 (33%)	ND (ND)	ND
Johannsson *et al.*[49]	97 (~40%)	ND (ND)	38 (~30%)	ND (ND)	0.45
Pharoah *et al.*[56]	552 (30%)	119 (19%)	127 (21%)	24 (25%)	0.005

NS, not significant; ND, not documented

SURGICAL PREVENTION

The woman seeking advice about prophylactic bilateral mastectomy and/or prophylactic bilateral salpingo-oophorectomy often feels misunderstood. She is confronted with the medical indications for prophylactic surgery, including family or personal history of breast cancer and/or ovarian cancer, multiple previous breast biopsies, unreliable results on physical examination because of nodular breasts, findings of dense breast tissue on X-ray mamography, mastodynia, ovarian cysts, insufficient screening modalities for ovarian cancer, and cancerphobia[60]. Her individual personal background and her fear related to breast and/or ovarian cancer cannot be quantified and evaluated on a routine basis. Therefore, physicians often misinterpret the wish for a definitive solution of her individual problem.

Studies about prophylactic bilateral mastectomy are not on a prospective basis. To date, only retrospective studies on bilateral prophylactic (subcutaneous) mastectomy have been published (Table 8). In women at risk, specific techniques of prophylactic breast surgery (simple, subcutaneous or complete mastectomy) and of reconstructive surgery are yet to be defined. Subcutaneous mastectomy may be not optimal for prophylaxis, because a substantial amount of breast tissue remains in the nipple–areolar complex. Three major studies have been published:

(1) Pennisi and Capozzi[61] (1500 women, 300 women having first-degree relatives with breast cancer, 15 years follow-up, six cases of breast cancer in women who had undergone a prophylactic mastectomy);

Table 8 Overview of studies with prophylactic bilateral mastectomy in patients at risk for breast cancer, and outcome

	Humphrey[75]	*Woods*[76]	*Bohmert*[77]	*Pennisi and Capozzi*[61]	*Hartmann et al.*[63]
Total no. of patients	285	1400	155	1500	639
No. (%) of high-risk patients*	16 (6%)	NS	90 (58%)	735 (49%)	214 (33%)
Mastectomy	subcutaneous	subcutaneous	simple	subcutaneous	subcutaneous
Median follow-up period (years)	ND	16–20	2	9	14
Total no. of patients who developed breast cancer	3	3	ND	6	7
Percentage of high-risk patients who developed breast cancer	19	ND	ND	0.81	1.4

*High-risk definition: patients with a positive breast cancer family history, *in situ* carcinomas or contralateral breast cancer. ND, not documented

(2) Ziegler and Kroll[62] (1500 women, 450 women having first-degree relatives with breast cancer, 9 years follow-up, 15 cases of breast cancer in women who had undergone a prophylactic mastectomy);

(3) Hartman and colleagues[63] (639 women, 214 women having a high and 425 having a moderate breast cancer risk, 14 years follow-up, four cases of breast cancer in women who had undergone a prophylactic mastectomy).

Only the Hartmann study provided sufficient details on the family history for a conclusive evaluation of the surgical effect[63]. According to the risk evaluation 37.5 women in the prophylactic bilateral mastectomy cohort were estimated to develop breast cancer, with the actual number being four cases of breast cancer (reduction in risk 89.5%; $p < 0.001$). For further evaluation, the women in the high-risk group ($n = 214$) were compared to their sisters, who did not undergo prophylactic surgery ($n = 403$). In the group of sisters without surgery, 156 (39%) cases of breast cancer were diagnosed, while in the high-risk group of women who had undergone prophylactic bilateral mastectomy, three breast cancer (1.4%) cases were identified (Table 8). Even though these data provide the best indication for a protective effect of prophylactic bilateral

Table 9 Overview of studies with prophylactic bilateral salpingo-oophorectomy in patients at risk for ovarian cancer, and outcome

	Tobacman et al.[64]	*Piver et al.*[65]	*Struewing et al./ NCI*[66]
Total no. of patients	28	324	44
No. (%) of high-risk patients*	28	324	44
Median follow-up period (years)	1–10	1–27	460 ps. ys.
Total no. of patients who developed cancer	3	6	2
Percentage of high-risk patients who developed cancer	11	2	4

*High-risk definition: patients with two first-degree relatives with ovarian cancer, or *BRCA1*- or *BRCA2*-positive women, or hysterectomy in the setting of an *HNPCC* germline mutation; ps. ys., person years

mastectomy, it has to be remembered that it is a retrospective study on a defined cohort, without genetic testing and using subcutaneous prophylactic bilateral mastectomy.

Three major studies concerning prophylactic bilateral salpingo-oophorectomy have been published[64–66]. Altogether, prophylactic bilateral salpingo-oophorectomy was performed in 396 high-risk patients because of their positive family history (Table 9). The highest risk after prophylactic bilateral salpingo-oophorectomy for these women appeared to be peritoneal carcinomatosis, which occurred in 11 patients (3%). This may be explained by any of the following:

(1) Occult ovarian cancer present at the time of surgery;

(2) Malignancy of ectopic ovarian tissue;

(3) Malignancy of the peritoneum, which is derived from celomic epithelium, the same embryological origin as the surface epithelium of the ovary.

Short- and long-term data on mortality due to prophylactic bilateral salpingo-oophorectomy are not available.

ANXIETY AND QUALITY OF LIFE

Members of high-risk breast cancer and/or ovarian cancer families develop anxiety, depression and fear of cancer[67]. These emotions accompany them from childhood onwards and may be highest at the age the youngest family member developed breast cancer and/or ovarian cancer. Many consultees seeking advice for preventive options or prophylactic bilateral mastectomy and/or prophylactic bilateral salpingo-oophorectomy have seen their relatives suffer and die from cancer at an early age. Sometimes this fear leads to a kind of cancerphobia and/or (extremely) inadequate lifestyle[67]. Because of the ineffective ovarian cancer screening modalities, there may be additional fear for members of ovarian cancer families. A descriptive study of reactions to *BRCA1* test results among 181 members of 14 *BRCA1* families showed that ten of 31 (32%) consultees in the *BRCA1*-positive category and 15 of 68 (22%) in the *BRCA1*-negative category had considered prophylactic bilateral mastectomy prior to their test results[67]. In contrast, 35% in the *BRCA1*-positive category contemplated prophylactic bilateral mastectomy after receiving their results, but none of the *BRCA1*-negative women continued to consider this option. Prior to the testing period, prophylactic bilateral mastectomy was performed in five of 57 (9%) *BRCA1*-positive and in seven of 78 (9%) *BRCA1*-negative women. Women who had negative *BRCA1* results after prophylactic bilateral mastectomy were still satisfied. They had made the best choice with the information available at the time of making their decision[67]. Women undergoing prophylactic bilateral mastectomy after adequate counselling do not regret their decision, but are relieved of the fear of cancer[68–70]. Their quality of life in the follow-up period is improved due to the lack of fear[67]. Furthermore, direct breast reconstruction surgery is not wanted by all women undergoing prophylactic bilateral mastectomy; some women refuse any breast reconstruction at all. This may be the psychological expression of the fact that the breast is seen as an organ of fear, and, after prophylactic bilateral mastectomy is carried out, this fear should completely disappear. Data on secondary reconstructive surgery are not yet available.

Women with familial ovarian cancer or *BRCA1/2* mutation carriers more often choose to undergo prophylactic bilateral salpingo-oophorectomy at a premenopausal age. This leads to undesirable menopausal symptoms (sweating, depression, sleep disturbances, early osteopenia, etc.), reducing the quality of life. These symptoms may disappear by using HRT, but the current controversy of HRT for women at increased risk for breast cancer may lead to insecurity.

CONCLUSION

To guarantee a comprehensive approach for women from high-risk families, they should be counselled in an interdisciplinary setting with experts on gynaecological oncology, human genetics and psychotherapy[13,24]. Only this setting provides the opportunity for the consultee to gather the most information she can with which to form her own opinion. In addition, consultees receive psychological support both prior to and after the process of decision-making. Risk assessment is variable, and medical interventions, screening and early-detection programs are the alternatives to be considered[13,14]. However, most recommendations for screening, early cancer detection and medical or surgical preventive measures are based on expert opinion[14] and not on prospective randomized trials or cohort studies.

Many indications point to clinical, pathological, endocrine and molecular differences between sporadic and inherited breast and ovarian cancer. The real susceptibility of gene mutation carriers for breast, ovarian and other cancers needs to be evaluated prospectively in a larger population. Further prospective randomized studies are needed to elucidate the pathological and endocrine features, as well as to establish environmental risk factors, which will all influence the clinical management of high-risk women and their decision regarding prophylactic surgery. Until these studies provide sufficient scientific bases for the decision whether or not to undergo prophylactic surgery, advice should be offered on an individual basis to the women seeking help regarding this important individual health issue.

ACKNOWLEDGEMENT

This work was supported by the Hereditary Breast and Ovarian Cancer Multicenter Trial, Deutsche Krebshilfe, Bonn, Germany.

REFERENCES

1. Bailar JC, Gornik HL. Cancer undefeated. *N Engl J Med* 1997;336:1569–74
2. Fearon ER. Human cancer syndromes: clues to the origin and nature of cancer. *Science* 1997;278:1043–50
3. Ford D, Easton DF, Stratton M, *et al.* Genetic heterogeneity and penetrance analysis of the *BRCA1* and *BRCA2* genes in breast cancer families. *Am J Hum Genet* 1998;62:676–89
4. Easton D, Ford D, Peto J. Inherited susceptibility to breast cancer. *Cancer Surv* 1993;18: 95–113
5. Narod SA, Goldgar D, Cannon-Albright L, *et al.* Risk modifiers in carriers of *BRCA1* mutations. *Int J Cancer* 1995;64:394–8
6. Easton D. Breast cancer genes – what are the real risks? *Nature Genet* 1997;17:210–11
7. Claus EB, Risch NJ, Thompson WD. Autosomal dominant inheritance of early-onset breast cancer. *Cancer* 1994;73:643–51
8. Schmidt S, Becher H, Chang-Claude J. Breast cancer risk assessment: use of complete pedigree information and the effect of misspecified ages at diagnosis of affected relatives. *Hum Genet* 1998;102:348–56

9. Lyman GH, Kuderer NM. Basic population and cancer genetics and their use in the assessment of cancer risk. *Eur J Cancer* 1997;33:2160–6
10. Wright JC, Weinstein MC. Gains in life expectancy from medical interventions – standardizing data on outcomes. *N Engl J Med* 1998;339:380–6
11. Schrag D, Kuntz KM, Garber JE, Weeks JC. Decision analysis – effects of prophylactic mastectomy and oophorectomy on life expectancy among women with *BRCA1* or *BRCA2* mutations. *N Engl J Med* 1997;336:1465–71
12. Grann VR, Panageas KS, Whang W, Antman KH, Neugut AI. Decision analysis of prophylactic mastectomy and oophorectomy in *BRCA1*-positive or *BRCA2*-positive patients. *J Clin Oncol* 1998;16:979–85
13. Beckmann MW, Schnuerch HG, Bodden-Heidrich R, *et al.* Early cancer detection programmes for women at high risk for breast and ovarian cancer: a proposal of practical guidelines. *Eur Cancer Prevent* 1996;5:468–75
14. Burke W, Daly M, Garber J, *et al.* Recommendations for follow-up care of individuals with inherited predisposition to cancer. *J Am Med Assoc* 1997;277:997–1003
15. Schulz KD, Duda V, Schreer I, Heywang-Koebrunner SH. Moeglichkeiten der Brustkrebsfrueherkennung. *Gynaekologe* 1997;30:631–6
16. Kerlikowske K, Grady D, Ernster V. Benefit of mammography screening in women aged 40–49 years: current evidence from randomized controlled trials. *Cancer* 1995;76: 1679–81
17. Elmore JG, Barton MB, Moceri VM, Polk S, Arena PJ, Fletcher SW. Ten-year risk of false positive screening mammograms and clinical breast examinations. *N Engl J Med* 1998;338: 1089–96
18. National Institutes of Health Consensus Development Panel. Special article. National Institutes of Health consensus development conference statement: breast cancer screening for women aged 40–49, January 21–23, 1997. *J Natl Cancer Inst* 1997;89:1015–26
19. Bick U. An integrated early detection concept in women with a genetic predisposition for breast cancer. *Radiology* 1997;37:591–6
20. Baines CJ, Vidmar M, McKeown-Eyssen G, Tibshirani R. Impact of menstrual phase on false-negative mammograms in the Canadian National Breast Screening Study. *Cancer* 1997;80:720–4
21. Law J. Cancers detected and induced in mammographic screening: new screening schedules and younger women with family history. *Br J Radiol* 1997;70;62–9
22. Bauer B, Veit R, Vogel E, Bernhardt JH. Bildgebende Diagnostik der weiblichen Brust. *Dtsch Aerztebl* 1997;94:A-2440–41
23. Beckmann MW, Untch M, Rabe T, Schulz KD, Bender HG. Chemoprävention des Mammakarzinoms. *Gynaekologe* 1999;32:150–7
24. Schmutzler RK, Kempe A, Kiechle M, Beckmann MW. Gegenwärtiger Stand der klinischen Beratung und Betreuung von Frauen mit einer erblichen Disposition für das Mammakarzinom. *Dtsch Med Wochenschr* 1999;124:563–6
25. Beckmann MW, Timmermann D. Gibt es ein Populations – oder ein Risikogruppenscreening für das Ovarialkarzinom? *Gynaekologe* 1997;30:85–91

26. DePriest PD, Gallion HH, Pavlik EJ, Kryscio RJ, van Nagell JR. Transvaginal sonography as a screening method for the detection of early ovarian cancer. *Gynecol Oncol* 1997;65:408–14
27. Goldberg JM, Piver MS, Mohannad FJ, Blumenson L. Age at onset of ovarian cancer in women with a strong family history of ovarian cancer. *Gynecol Oncol* 1997;66:3–9
28. Fisher B, Constantino JP, Wickerham L, *et al.* Tamoxifen for prevention of breast cancer: report of the National Surgical Adjuvant Breast and Bowel Project P-1 Study. *J Natl Cancer Inst* 1998;90:1371–88
29. Powels T, Eeles R, Ashley S, *et al.* Interim analysis of the incidence of breast cancer in the Royal Marsden Hospital Tamoxifen Randomised Chemoprevention Trial. *Lancet* 1998; 352:98–101
30. Veronesi U, Maisonneuve P, Costa A, *et al.* Prevention of breast cancer with tamoxifen: preliminary findings from the Italian Randomized Trial Among Hysterectomized Women. *Lancet* 1998;352:93–7
31. Claus EB, Risch N, Thompson WD. Autosomal dominant inheritance of early-onset breast cancer. Implications for risk prediction. *Cancer* 1994;73:643–51
32. Whittemore AS, Harris R, Intyre J and the Collaborative Ovarian Cancer Group. Characteristics relating to ovarian cancer risk: collaborative analysis of 12 US case–control studies. II. Invasive epithelial ovarian cancers in white women. *Am J Epidemiol* 1992;136: 1184–203
33. Beral V, Hermon C, Kay C, Hannaford P, Darby S, Reeves G. Mortality associated with oral contraceptive use: 25 years follow up of cohort of 46 000 women from Royal College of General Practitioners Oral Contraceptive Study. *Br Med J* 1999;318:96–100
34. Narod S, Risch H, Moslehi R, *et al.* Oral contraceptive use reduces the risk of hereditary ovarian cancer. *N Engl J Med* 1998;339:424–8
35. Collaborative Group on Hormonal Factors in Breast Cancer. Breast cancer and hormonal contraceptives: collaborative reanalysis of individual data on 53 297 women with breast cancer and 100 239 women without breast cancer from 54 epidemiological studies. *Lancet* 1996;347:1713–27
36. Brinton LA, Daling JR, Liff JM, *et al.* Oral contraceptives and breast cancer risk among younger women. *J Natl Cancer Inst* 1995;87:827–35
37. Ursin G, Henderson BE, Haile RW, *et al.* Does oral contraceptive use increase the risk of breast cancer in women with *BRCA1/2* mutations? *Cancer Res* 1997;57:3678–81
38. Gaffney DK, Brohet RM, Lewis CM, *et al.* Response to radiation therapy and prognosis in breast cancer patients with *BRCA1* and *BRCA2* mutations. *Radiother Oncol* 1998;47: 129–36
39. Verhoog LC, Brekelmans CTM, Seynaeve C, *et al.* Survival and tumor characteristics of breast cancer patients with germline mutations of *BRCA1*. *Lancet* 1998;361:316–21
40. Ansquer Y, Gautier C, Fourquet A, Asselain B, Stoppa-Lyonnet D. Survival in early-onset *BRCA1* breast-cancer patients. *Lancet* 1998;352:541
41. Robson M, Gilewski T, Haas B, *et al.* *BRCA*-associated breast cancer in young women. *J Clin Oncol* 1998;16:1642–9
42. Johannsson O, Loman N, Borg A, Olsson H. Pregnancy-associated breast cancer in *BRCA1* and *BRCA2* germline mutation carriers. *Lancet* 1998;352:1359–60

43. Claus EB, Risch N, Thompson WD, Carter D. Relationship between breast histopathology and family history of breast cancer. *Cancer* 1993;71:147–53
44. Marcus JN, Watson P, Page DL, *et al.* Hereditary breast cancer. Pathology, prognosis, and *BRCA1* and *BRCA2* gene linkage. *Cancer* 1996;77:697–709
45. Lagios MD, Rose MR, Margolin FR. Tubular carcinoma of the breast: association with multicentricity, bilaterality, and family history of mammary carcinoma. *Am J Clin Pathol* 1980;73:25–30
46. Breast Cancer Linkage Consortium. Pathology of familial breast cancer: differences between breast cancers in carriers of *BRCA1* or *BRCA2* mutations and sporadic cases. *Lancet* 1997;349:1505–10
47. Lakhani S, Jacquemier J, Sloane JP, *et al.* Multifactorial analysis of differences between sporadic breast cancers and cancers involving *BRCA1* and *BRCA2* mutations. *J Natl Cancer Inst* 1998;90:1138–45
48. Eisinger F, Jacquemier J, Charpin C, *et al.* Mutations at *BRCA1*: the medullary breast carcinoma revisited. *Cancer Res* 1998;58:1588–92
49. Johannsson O, Idvall I, Anderson C, *et al.* Tumor biological features of *BRCA1*-induced breast and ovarian cancer. *Eur J Cancer* 1997;33:362–71
50. Petersson C, Pandis N, Mertens F, *et al.* Chromosome aberrations in prophylactic mastectomies from women belonging to breast cancer families. *Genes Chromosomes Cancer* 1996;16:185–8
51. Osin P, Gusterson BA, Philp E, *et al.* Predicted anti-oestrogen resistance in *BRCA*-associated familial breast cancers. *Eur J Cancer* 1998;34:1683–6
52. Teixeira MR, Pandis N, Gerdes AM, *et al.* Cytogenetic abnormalities in an *in situ* ductal carcinoma and five prophylactically removed breasts from members of family with hereditary breast cancer. *Breast Cancer Res Treat* 1996;38:177–82
53. Tirkkonen M, Johannsson O, Agnarsson BA, *et al.* Distinct somatic genetic changes associated with tumor progression in carriers of *BRCA1* and *BRCA2* germ-line mutations. *Cancer Res* 1997;57:1222–7
54. Ingvarsson S, Geirsdottir EK, Johannesdottir G, *et al.* High incidence of loss of heterozygosity in breast tumors from carriers of the *BRCA2* 999del5 mutation. *Cancer Res* 1998;58:4421–5
55. Lerman C, Hughes C, Lemon SJ, *et al.* What you don't know can hurt you: adverse psychologic effects in members of *BRCA1*-linked and *BRCA2*-linked families who decline genetic testing. *J Clin Oncol* 1998;16:1650–4
56. Pharoah PD, Easton DF, Stockton DL, Gayther S, Ponder BA. Survival in familial, *BRCA1*-associated, and *BRCA2*-associated epithelial ovarian cancer. *Cancer Res* 1999;59: 868–71
57. Salazar H, Godwin AK, Daly MB, *et al.* Microscopic benign and invasive malignant neoplasms and a cancer prone phenotype in prophylactic oophorectomies. *J Natl Cancer Inst* 1996;88:1810–20
58. Werness BA, Afify AM, Bielat KL, Eltabbakh GH, Piver MS, Paterson JM. Altered surface and cyst epithelium of ovaries removed prophylactically from women with a family history of ovarian cancer. *Hum Pathol* 1999;30:151–7

59. Stratton JF, Buckley CH, Lowe D, Ponder BA. Comparison of prophylactic oophorectomy specimens from carriers and noncarriers of *BRCA1* or *BRCA2* gene mutation. *J Natl Cancer Inst* 1999;91:626–8
60. Hoskins KF, Stopfer JE, Calzone KA, *et al.* Assessment and counseling for women with family history of breast cancer. *J Am Med Assoc* 1995;273:577–85
61. Pennisi VR, Capozzi A. Subcutaneous mastectomy data: a final statistical analysis of 1500 patients. *Aesthetic Plast Surg* 1989;13:15–21
62. Ziegler LD, Kroll SS. Primary breast cancer after prophylactic mastectomy. *Am J Clin Oncol* 1991;14:451–4
63. Hartmann LC, Schaid DJ, Woods JE, *et al.* Efficacy of bilateral prophylactic mastectomy in women with family history of breast cancer. *N Engl J Med* 1999;340:77–84
64. Tobacman JK, Greene MH, Tucker MA, Costa J, Kase R, Fraumeni JF. Intra-abdominal carcinomatosis after prophylactic oophorectomy in ovarian-cancer-prone families. *Lancet* 1982;2:795–7
65. Piver SM, Jishi MF, Tsukada Y, Nava G. Primary peritoneal carcinoma after prophylactic oophorectomy in women with a family history of ovarian cancer. *Cancer* 1993;71:2751–5
66. Struewing JP, Watson P, Easton DF, Ponder BAJ, Lynch HT, Tucker MA. Prophylactic oophorectomy in inherited breast/ovarian cancer families. *Monogr Natl Cancer Inst* 1995;17:33–5
67. Lynch HT, Lemon SJ, Durham C, *et al.* A descriptive study of *BRCA1* testing and reactions to disclosure of test results. *Cancer* 1997;79:2219–28
68. Klijn JGM, Janin N. Current Controversies in Cancer. Should prophylactic surgery be used in women with a high risk of breast cancer? *Eur J Cancer* 1997;33:2149–59
69. Steel CM. Implications of studies of inherited predisposition for prevention and treatment. In Ponder BAJ, Waring MJ, eds. *The Genetics of Cancer.* Dordrecht: Kluwer Academic Publishers, 1995:159–75
70. Stefanek ME, Helzlsouer KH, Wilcox PM, Anp CS, Houn F. Predictors of and satisfaction with bilateral prophylactic mastectomy. *Prev Med* 1995;24:412–19
71. Buller RE, Anderson B, Connor JP, Robinson R. Familial ovarian cancer. *Gynecol Oncol* 1993;51:160–6
72. Chang J, Fryatt I, Ponder BA, Fisher C, Gore ME. A matched control study of familial epithelial ovarian cancer: patient characteristics, response to chemotherapy and outcome. *Ann Oncol* 1995;6:80–2
73. Rubin SC, Benjamin I, Behbakht K, *et al.* Clinical and pathological features of ovarian cancer in women with germline mutations of *BRCA1*. *N Engl J Med* 1996;335:1413–16
74. Brunet JS, Narod SA, Tonin P, Foulkes WD. *BRCA1* mutations and survival in women with ovarian cancer. *N Engl J Med* 1997;336:1256
75. Humphrey LJ. Subcutaneous mastectomy is not a prophylaxis against carcinoma of the beast: opinion and knowledge? *Am J Surg* 1983;145:311–12
76. Woods JE. Breast reconstruction: current state of the art. *Mayo Clin Proc* 1986;61:579–85
77. Bohmert HH. Subcutaneous mastectomy. In Grundfest-Broniatowski S, Esselstyn CB Jr, eds. *Controversies in Breast Disease: Diagnosis and Management.* New York: Marcel Dekker, 1988:235–59

13

Histogenic classification of Fallopian tube tumors with clinical and pathological reminders

R. Nappi and L. Nappi

INTRODUCTION

Neoplastic pathology of the Fallopian tube is a rare condition, unreported in childhood, representing a minimal percentage (0.3%) of all gynecological tumors. Malignancies are by far more frequent than benign lesions (Table 1). Primary malignant tumors represent one-tenth of the secondary tumors which propagate from ovarian, endometrial and extragenital sites (stomach, intestine, pancreas)[1]. A tubal metastatic implant secondary to mucoid gastric carcinoma, a true Krukenberg tumor, is known to exist. The rarity of the primary tubal tumor has caused the organ to be considered of low oncogenic capacity, as opposed to its well-known vulnerability to infections. Benign and malignant tubal tumors originate from:

(1) Any one of the three anatomical tunicae that form the tubal wall (mucosa, muscularis, serosa);

(2) Embryonic remnants;

(3) Tissues extrinsic to the salpinx uterina.

Table 1 Types of tubal tumor

(1)	Tumors originating from the endosalpinx (tunica mucosa)
(2)	Tumors originating from the myosalpinx (tunica muscularis)
(3)	Tumors originating from the tubal serosa (tunica serosa)
(4)	Cysts and tumors originating from embryonic remnants
	(a) Müllerian
	(b) Wolffian
	(c) Mesothelial
(5)	Tumors of the salpinx uterina originating from extrinsic tissues
	(a) Ovary
	(b) Trophoblast
(6)	Pseudotumors

ENDOSALPINX

Polyp

This tumor is evidenced by hysterosalpingography, hysteroscopy and the examination of operative specimens. It is a small formation with a wide base, often bilateral. It has an adenomatous structure deriving from ectopic endometrium and is lined by tubal epithelium containing mucoid ciliated cells[2].

Papilloma

Papillomas are less frequently observed than tubal polyps and are usually found in the medial portion of the tube. Like the tubal polyp, a papilloma may cause subfertility. It has a structure comprising delicate branching of connective tissue covered by a flattened, monolayer epithelium without cilia. It is not thought to be related to tubal cancer.

Carcinoma

Carcinoma of the endosalpinx is a rare malignancy with an unfavorable prognosis. It has a reported incidence of 0.24–1.11% of all gynecological cancers. To date, approximately 1200 cases have been reported in the literature, with an annual increase calculated to be approximately 20 new cases. The age of incidence ranges from 39 to 80 years in recent studies and 19–85 years by analyzing larger series[3]. Carcinoma of the endosalpinx has the highest frequency of all tubal malignancies. It is bilateral in 26% of cases and spreads by direct extension into the peritoneum. It is a poorly differentiated tumor and is easily recognized as being malignant. The carcinoma has a papillary alveolar structure with fibrovascular stalks and is lined by epithelium resembling normal endosalpinx. Variants are clear-cell, endometrioid and adenosquamous forms[4]. Intraepithelial carcinoma and adenomatous hyperplasia of the endosalpinx have been observed. A distinctive sign is its fusiform swelling, involving two-thirds or the entire length of the tube. The classical clinical triad includes lower abdominal pain, vaginal bleeding and leukorrhea, and laterouterine tumor mass. There is rarely correct preoperative diagnosis[5]. The value of vaginal cytology for diagnosis is controversial; it has been reported to contribute to the diagnosis in 10–60% of cases[6,7]. Nuclear magnetic resonance, computerized axial tomography, sonography, hysterosalpingography, celioscopy, lymphography and antigen CA 125 are dissimilar in their diagnostic importance. One major difficulty is the low diagnostic suspect index for this rare disease, so that generic signs of pelvic malignancy attract more attention for organs with a high neoplastic incidence, such as the ovary, than for the Fallopian tube. From the prognostic point of view, in addition to the definite importance of a tumor in an advanced stage, minor predictors have been reported to be the absence of closure of the fimbriated extremity of the tube and an age over 66 years[8]. Different methods of staging tubal carcinoma are known, one of which is based on criteria that evaluate the degree of histological differentiation, depth of infiltration, bilaterality and diffusion[9]. Despite the difference in structure between the ovary (parenchymal) and the Fallopian tube (musculomembranous), the International Federation of Gynaecology and Obstetrics staging system used in epithelial cancer of the ovary is also utilized in tubal cancer.

The treatment has not been well defined and in general it conforms to the same patterns followed in ovarian cancer. Minimal surgical management is considered to be total hysterectomy, bilateral salpingo-oophorectomy and omentectomy. Contraindicated are local excision and simple salpingectomy for frequent contralateral and/or uterine involvement. Chemotherapy is with carboplatin–cisplatin singly or in association with other agents. Radiotherapy is carried out by pelvic irradiation, abdominal bath and intraperitoneal isotope ^{32}P. Actuarial 3-year survival rate is 52% for Stage I disease, 50% for Stage II and 6% for Stages III and IV disease.

Malignant mixed müllerian tumor

This is a rare sarcomatous neoplasia, representing less than 1% of all genital sarcomas[10]. Two histological forms are known: first, the homologous variant, in which the tumor reproduces various components of the müllerian tract such as fibrous connective tissue stroma, glands and smooth muscle; second, the heterologous variant, which is made of elements extrinsic to the müllerian tract, such as rhabdomyoblast or cartilage and bones, and is a typical neoplasm of childhood. The tumor is also found rarely in the corpus uteri, cervix, vagina, ovary and bladder[11].

Its rapid systemic hematogenous spread suggests aggressive treatment from the early stages of the disease. Approximately 30 cases have been reported in the literature.

MYOSALPINX

Leiomyoma

This is a rather small, infrequent tumor, unlike its uterine variety. It may also originate from the vascular walls in the isthmic portion and less frequently in the ampulla.

Leiomyosarcoma

This tumor is even more uncommon than leiomyoma and has a very poor prognosis. It spreads by direct extension and systemic hematogenous metastases. The tumor has spindle-shaped cells with atypical nuclei and a high mitotic index.

TUBAL SEROSA

Inclusion cysts

These are also called inflammatory cysts because they originate from peritubal adhesions. Their dimensions may vary from a few millimeters to several centimeters. They have a serous content. The cyst wall is lined with flat, mesothelial-type cells and may occasionally undergo metaplastic changes.

Walthard's inclusions

Walthard's inclusions are small, greyish-yellow plaques, 0.5–1.0 cm in diameter, disseminated on the tube and broad ligament. They may be confused with miliary tuberculosis. These inclusions arise from the microinvagination of ovarian mesothelial cells in metaplastic evolution.

Benign mesothelioma (adenomatous tumor)

This is the most frequent benign tubal tumor. Because of the peculiar histological structure, it has been variously described as lymphangioma, reticuloendothelioma, mesonephroma, lymphangiectatic myoma and even low-grade adenocarcinoma. Its postulated vascular or epithelial origin was never reliably evidenced in the past and therefore the simply descriptive name of adenomatoid tumor was used. The mesothelial origin is now well demonstrated and the appropriate name of benign mesothelioma is currently used. It is characterized by subserous yellowish-grey, firm, discrete nodules that occupy the myosalpinx, rarely exceeding 3 cm in diameter. Microscopically, solid cords and small oblong polygonal cavities are lined by flattened endothelial-looking cells or by large and vacuolated epithelial- or mesothelial-looking cells. This lesion is also frequent in the male (on the epididymis, testicular tunicae and spermatic cord). Simple surgical excision ensures recovery and recurrence is rare.

Endosalpingiosis

Endosalpingiosis consists of small serosal implants, histologically resembling tubal epithelium, that are also found on the peritoneum of the uterus, colon, rectosigmoid and mesosalpinx, and on the omentum, mainly in young women with chronic salpingitis, hydrosalpinx or tubal pregnancy. In rare cases it presents as a clinically or grossly evident mass that can be confused with a neoplasm[12,13]. Cells lining the implants are either flat or cuboidal with tuft-like structures, glands and occasional concentric microcalcifications. The histological similarity with the epithelium of some superficial ovarian cysts has linked the origin of such cysts to endosalpingiosis. Association with ovarian malignancies may engender diagnostic confusion with metastatic diffusion and cause perplexity as to the magnitude of surgery.

The origin has been variously ascribed to müllerian tissue, shedding of tubal epithelium, and metaplastic proliferation of the mesothelial or celomic epithelium. Endosalpingiosis may rarely undergo malignant transformation. Pelvic pain has been pointed out as an important clinical feature[14].

CYSTS AND TUMORS ORIGINATING FROM EMBRYONIC REMNANTS

Paratubal cysts

The majority of these lesions are of either paramesonephric müllerian or mesothelial origin. Few are of mesonephric wolffian origin. The secretory and ciliated cells of the paramesonephric system produce intracystic fluid, distension of the lumen and cyst formation. In contrast, low cuboidal mesonephric epithelium has minimal secretory activity and is enfolded in a firm muscle that allows little potential for the formation of cysts. These cysts are unilocular, thin walled, seldom bilateral and are usually small in size (< 5 cm), but may reach large dimensions (> 10 cm), filling the whole abdomen[15]. Paratubal cysts may occasionally exhibit the microscopic pattern of a low-grade malignancy, with hypercellularity and complex papillate formations, in which case possible secondary diffusion of ovarian or distant primary tumor must be ruled out.

Mesothelial paramesonephric cysts are clinically silent except in acute complications. Surgery is mandatory due to the risk of malignant transformation in cystadenocarcinoma. Their resection may involve surgical separation from a pelvic ureter and major pelvic blood vessels.

Pedunculated hydatid of Morgagni

This is a müllerian vestige, residual to the celomic invagination at the time of formation of the müllerian duct, or, like the fimbria, it derives from accessory tubal lumina or may represent the dilated distal end of Gartner's duct. Pedunculated hydatid of Morgagni is asymptomatic, 1–4 cm in size and well known to surgeons and endoscopists. It is devoid of evolutional complications and therefore the hydatid can be safely left undisturbed, although nothing is easier than fastening a ligature around its base and removing it.

Mesosalpingian tumors

These are solid, encapsulated tumors, varying in size from 1.3 to 13.0 cm. Histologically, they show solid areas or tubular sertoli-like structures, or may resemble adenomatoid tumors. Electron microscopic features indicate that they originate from wolffian structures[16].

TUBAL TUMORS ORIGINATING FROM EXTRINSIC TISSUES

Benign cystic teratoma (dermoid)

Although extremely uncommon, dermoid cysts are more frequent than solid teratomas. Histologically, they are similar to both mature ovarian teratomas (skin, muscle and bone derivatives) and functioning ovarian tumors. Hormone-producing tubal teratomas may partially or totally consist of thyroid tissue and form a struma salpingii, with clinical signs of hyperthyroidism. Tubal dermoids originate from ectopic ovarian components (accessory ovary) or from primordial germ cells arrested during migration from the yolk sac to the gonad. Benign cystic teratoma is usually unilateral, pedunculated and small; it only rarely enlarges up to 20 cm in diameter. Malignant transformation and intraperitoneal rupture has been reported. Concomitant ipsilateral or contralateral pregnancy is possible. Fertility is not impaired: 19 out of 24 women aged 25–55 years who were operated on for salpingian teratoma were reported to have had normal pregnancies[17,18] Other additional tubal tumors originating from ovarian tissue include dysgerminoma and granulosa-cell tumor.

Choriocarcinoma and hydatidiform mole

Choriocarcinomatous transformation of tubal pregnancy is a rare and threatening disease. Overall, the incidence of tubal localization of choriocarcinoma ranges from 0.65 to 5.0%. The histogenesis is unclear. Orthotopic choriocarcinoma starts in a primary tubal pregnancy; in heterotopic choriocarcinoma, extrauterine pregnancy is secondary to an intrauterine gestation diffused to the salpinx by embolic transportation of chorionic villi[19]. It has been postulated that the tumor may be independent of pregnancy and may start in a tube with teratogenic changes. Choriocarcinoma of the salpinx is reported to be more frequent than tubal hydatidiform mole. However, in contrast to uterine choriocarcinoma, the tubal tumor is not preceded by the hydatidiform mole and consequently simple linear salpingotomy would be safe treatment for hydatidiform mole occurring in the ampullary portion[20]. Salpingian choriocarcinoma reproduces all histological molar patterns, such as rich trophoblastic proliferation and very immature appearance of the syncytiotrophoblast. Evolution, progression and treatment comply with the uterine form. Mortality rate ranges from 85 to 93%, but more recently the 5-year survival rate is reported to be around 65%, owing to chemotherapy. Histological examination of tubal pregnancy specimens is a very important prophylactic standard.

PSEUDOTUMORS

Under this heading come small nodular thickenings or non-neoplastic salpingian implants, which are usually diagnosed as endometriosis, adenomyosis or salpingitis isthmicanodosa.

REFERENCES

1. Ng P, Lawton F. Fallopian tube carcinoma – a review. *Ann Acad Med Singapore* 1998;27:693–7
2. Lisa GR, Gioia JD, Rubin IC. Observation on the interstitial portion of the Fallopian tube. *Gynecol Obstet* 1954;99:159–64
3. Butler DF, Bolton ME, Spanos WJ Jr, *et al.* Retrospective analysis of patients with primary Fallopian tube carcinoma treated at the University of Louisville. *J Ky Med Assoc* 1999;97:154–64
4. Rabczynski J, Ziolkowski P, Kochman A, *et al.* Primary Fallopian tube carcinoma. Histopathology of 46 cases. *Pol J Pathol* 1998;49:285–92
5. Sedlis A. Carcinoma of the Fallopian tube. *Surg Clin North Am* 1978;58:121–9
6. Takashina T, Ito E, Kudo R. Cytologic diagnosis of primary tubal cancer. *Acta Cytol* 1985;29:367–72
7. Hirai Y, Chen JT, Hamada T, *et al.* Clinical and cytologic aspects of primary Fallopian tube carcinoma. *Acta Cytol* 1987;31:834–40

8. Alvarado-Cabrero I, Young RH, Vamvakas EC, *et al.* Carcinoma of the Fallopian tube: a clinicopathological study of 105 cases with observations on staging and prognostic factors. *Gynecol Oncol* 1999;72:367–79
9. Shiller HM, Silvergerg SG. Staging and prognosis in primary carcinoma of the Fallopian tube. *Cancer* 1971;28:389–402
10. Ebert AD, Perez-Canto A, Schaller G, *et al.* Stage I primary malignant mixed müllerian tumor of the Fallopian tube. Report of a case with five-year survival after minimal surgery without adjuvant treatment. *J Reprod Med* 1998;43:598–600
11. Buchwalter CL, Jenison EL, Fromm M, *et al.* Pure embryonal rhabdomyosarcoma of the Fallopian tube. *Gynecol Oncol* 1997;67:95–101
12. Clement PB, Young RH. Florid cystic endosalpingiosis with tumor-like manifestations: a report of four cases including the first reported cases of transmural endosalpingiosis of the uterus. *Am J Surg Pathol* 1999;23:166–75
13. Zinsser KR, Wheeler JE. Endosalpingiosis in the omentum: a study of autopsy and surgical material. *Am J Surg Pathol* 1982;6:109–13
14. Laufer MR, Heerema AE, Parsons KE, *et al.* Endosalpingiosis: clinical presentation and follow-up. *Gynecol Obstet Invest* 1998;46:195–8
15. Samara M, Woodruff D. Paratubal cysts: frequency, histogenesis and associated clinical features. *Obstet Gynecol* 1985;65:691–6
16. Wagatsuma S, Yaegashi N, Namiki T, *et al.* A case of female adnexal tumor of probable wolffian origin: histologically, tumor cells showed three different patterns. *Tohoku J Exp Med* 1997;181:371–7
17. Massouda D, Wortham GF, Oakley JL. Tubal pregnancy associated with a benign cystic teratoma of the Fallopian tube. *J Reprod Med* 1988;24:563–9
18. Hseih CS, Cheng GF, Liu YG, *et al.* Benign cystic teratoma of unilateral Fallopian tube associated with intrauterine pregnancy: a case report. *Chung Hua I Hsueh Tsa Chih (Taipei)* 1998;61:239–42
19. Su YN, Cheng WF, Chen CA, *et al.* Pregnancy with primary tubal placental site trophoblastic tumor – a case report and literature review. *Gynecol Oncol* 1999;73:322–5
20. Newcomer JR. Ampullary tubal hydatidiform mole treated with linear salpingotomy. A case report. *J Reprod Med* 1998;43:913–15

Pelvic pain

14

Conscious pain mapping: pain evaluation at laparoscopy under local anesthesia in women with chronic pelvic pain

P. Reginald, L. Iyer and R. Fell

INTRODUCTION

Chronic pelvic pain is a common presenting complaint, but the cause of this symptom often remains undiagnosed. However, endometriosis, pelvic congestion, adhesions involving residual ovaries and ovarian remnants, chronic pelvic inflammatory disease, entrapment of the ilio-inguinal/hypogastric nerve and irritable bowel syndrome are some of the well-recognized causes of chronic pelvic pain. A good medical history and examination are useful in arriving at a diagnosis. Pelvic pain, deep dyspareunia, infertility and dysmenorrhea are characteristic symptoms of endometriosis, although up to 22% of women with this condition remain entirely asymptomatic. Women with ovarian remnant syndrome complain of cyclical pelvic pain, despite a history of having undergone bilateral oophorectomy, often carried out for extensive endometriosis or pelvic inflammatory disease. The diagnosis could be made by the finding of a follicle stimulating hormone level in the premenopausal range, indicating the presence of an active ovarian remnant whose enlargement in response to clomiphene could be monitored by ultrasound scanning. Women with residual ovary syndrome complain of deep dyspareunia, and examination typically reveals an enlarged, tender ovary that is often fixed to the vault. Chronic pain caused by the entrapment of the ilio-inguinal/hypogastric nerve is felt at the incision site, often radiating to the labia and the inner aspect of the thigh. Physical activity aggravates the pain and there is evidence of hyperesthesia in the inguinal region. Pain relief after the injection of local anesthetic

(0.5% bupivacaine) into the area is diagnostic. Patients with irritable bowel syndrome are usually polysymptomatic, but have symptoms predominantly affecting bowel function. This differentiates women with pelvic congestion, who are always in the reproductive age group with complaints relating to the pelvic organs. These symptoms include congestive dysmenorrhea (66%), deep dyspareunia (77%) and post-coital ache (66%). The symptoms of post-coital ache and a positive ovarian point tenderness (77%) are characteristic of women with pelvic congestion.

OBJECTIVE

Diagnostic laparoscopy is an established investigation for chronic pelvic pain, as it enables adequate visualization of the pelvic organs and identifies abnormalities. Many women with chronic pelvic pain, however, demonstrate no obvious pathology at laparoscopy. Moreover, the pathology noted at laparoscopy is not always the cause of the pain. Hence, some women continue to have pain, despite previous medical or surgical intervention, and multiple laparoscopic examinations are therefore not uncommon in these women. A precise diagnosis of the cause of the pain may be possible if an interactive approach with the patient is used at laparoscopy. The objective of our study was to locate the source and assess reproducibility of the pelvic pain at laparoscopy performed under local anesthesia (conscious pain mapping).

METHODS

A total of 43 women (mean age 33 years), with chronic pelvic pain of more than 6 months' duration, were recruited for laparoscopy under local anesthesia. The aims of the study and the procedure were explained to the patients and written informed consent was obtained. Patients were counselled in detail regarding the procedural events, such as the sensation of abdominal distension and head-down tilt, and the operating theatre environment. Obesity (body mass index > 30) was felt to be a relative contraindication to the procedure, as was surgical phobia, psychiatric disease or manifest anxiety. No premedication was given.

Anesthetic technique

The anesthesia involved a combination of an intravenous anxiolytic and opioid medication, along with local anesthetic at the trocar sites. Alternating doses of midazolam 70 μg/kg and pethidine 500 μg/kg were given intravenously and repeated at 5–10-min intervals if required. No more than two doses were required for any of the patients in the study. After infiltrating the skin, the deeper layers of tissue in the subumbilical area were thoroughly anesthetized using 20 ml of 0.25% bupivacaine with adrenaline 1 : 200 000. This area was infiltrated in a fan-shaped manner using a spinal needle.

Insertion of the laparoscope

A small incision was made transversely below the umbilicus. The patient was asked to protrude her abdominal wall and the Verre's needle was introduced simultaneously. A total of 1.5 l of nitrous oxide was insufflated intraperitoneally. The trocar and cannula were then inserted as the patient protruded her abdominal wall as before. All laparoscopies were performed by the senior author (PWR) using an Olympus 5.5-mm telescope with a 0° lens (A5290A). Illumination was provided by a 250-W, high-intensity cold light source and the images were viewed on a high-resolution color monitor using a chip camera. The suprapubic area was then infiltrated with 20 ml of 1% lignocaine in order to obtain immediate anesthesia for the insertion of the second trocar. After infiltrating the skin and subcutaneous tissue, the needle was advanced until it reached the peritoneum. Adequate infiltration of the peritoneum was made under direct vision with the laparoscope and the second trocar was then introduced. The cervix was not dilated and no intrauterine manipulation was carried out. The uterus was manipulated digitally or by using a sponge on a holding forceps in the vagina.

Pain mapping

The operator was blind to the exact side on which the patient experienced pain. A probe was introduced through the second cannula, and the intestines, uterus, tubes, ovaries and round ligaments were mobilized systematically. Adhesions, if present, were stretched and any pathological lesions, such as endometriosis, varicosities or ovarian cysts, were touched. This procedure will hitherto be referred to as probing.

The patient was instructed to score the discomfort experienced on probing on a verbal rating scale of 0–10. In addition, she was also asked whether such probing reproduced the pain that she complained of. The patients were invited to look at the monitor if they desired. They were not, however, orientated to the site or side of the organs being probed. Any pathological finding was always probed last. The entire pelvis was mapped twice for consistency of results.

RESULTS

Laparoscopic diagnosis of pelvic pathology was made in 18 and pelvic congestion in 13 patients and in eight women the pelvis was judged to be normal. In three women the procedure was considered to be unsatisfactory and in one the procedure was abandoned. In six of the 18 women with pathology, the pain was not reproduced by probing the area of abnormality. In six of the women with pelvic congestion, pain was confined to the uterus only, while in others the ovaries were also found to be tender. No site of pain was located in three of the women with a normal pelvis.

CONCLUSION

The pain was reproduced and the site identified in 35 of the 39 women who had a successful laparoscopy. This study demonstrates that the observed pathology was not the cause of pain in six out of 18 patients. In women with pelvic congestion, hysterectomy without bilateral salpingo-oophorectomy may be appropriate in cases where the pain is confined to the uterus only. Even in those women where the pelvis was judged to be normal, the site of pain was identified in five patients.

Postgraduate training

15

Training in obstetrics and gynaecology – the trainee's opinion

F. Nunes

INTRODUCTION

In 1975, the European Union of Medical Specialists participated in the development of the definition of the European Medical Directives. These Directives regulate the free movement of doctors and the mutual recognition of medical credentials throughout the European Community. These two aspects brought about the obligation of creating a European consensus on training programs, training centers and quality assurance.

Training in obstetrics and gynaecology in Europe is still quite heterogeneous, reflecting cultural, social and ethical differences. Nevertheless, many countries do seem to be approaching a standard; for example, the duration of training is now fairly uniform. The definition and recommendations on what is basic and should be common to all countries will help to achieve quality control in training.

Quality control should be centered on the training process and should take into account the following four aspects on which the quality of the final product (the specialist) depends: training program, training center, trainers and trainee.

TRAINING PROGRAMS

The changing of training programs involves structural modifications and significant costs. It is important to start with very simple and consensus determinations, that could be easily accepted and included in the training programs of all the European countries.

A clear definition should be made of what is required of a specialist in obstetrics and gynaecology. All training programs should have a syllabus of specific objectives in terms of knowledge, skill and attitudes for the various fields, with clearly defined targets. The trainee should be involved in all aspects of the training process.

To guarantee quality of training, quantification with minimum requirements is not compulsory, but it may be a step towards harmonization and quality improvement.

TRAINING CENTERS

It is essential that training takes place exclusively in training centers accredited by competent authorities. This will bring obvious direct implications for quality improvement. It will establish a list of recognized European training centers, and the number of trainees will be determined in accordance with the capacity of each department. This will increase the individual training quality.

The system of visits will allow detection and correction of deficiencies, both in organization and in equipment, installations and medical staff. We hope that this system will allow the participation of representatives of trainees (national or European commissions) in the visits to the departments. If we want to have any feedback on the training system, the opinion of the trainees should be relevant in attributing accreditation.

TRAINERS

While all specialists should be involved in the supervision of trainees, only some of them will be interested in, and will have the personal characteristics necessary, to take on the additional responsibilities of teaching. It is necessary to select the most capable teachers, but also to chose those that are more interested in teaching.

The adoption of criteria for selection of trainers, with protected teaching time and training in educational methods, will obviously promote a better quality of training. Courses for medical trainers, would also promote communication between European trainers and would facilitate harmonization.

ASSESSMENT

Few countries have a formal, final examination, while the standards of most countries rely on other forms of assessment. We all agree that all future specialists should be formally evaluated.

Independent of the method adopted by each country, two requirements should be made of any kind of assessment: it should assess knowledge, skills and attitudes; and it should permit, in time, the correction of the deficiencies detected in the training.

We think that high standards are best obtained by a well-structured tutor system with regular forms of assessment during training: self-assessment, formative assessment and summative assessment.

The recommendation for an official, common log book will help in the comparison of the results obtained in training in the different countries. Harmonization of standards with a certain flexibility of programs could be the strategy for success.

CONCLUSIONS

The European Network of Trainees in Obstetrics and Gynaecology (ENTOG) was created in 1996, to establish communication and represent the European trainees. the aims of ENTOG are to promote a better understanding of training in obstetrics and gynaecology in Europe, thus ensuring comparable and high standards of training.

The position of the European Board and College of Obstetrics and Gynaecology (EBCOG) working in co-operation with the National Authorities of each country and the trainees was an important step in allowing the establishment of common European recommendations for training. It is unlikely that complete harmonization of training in obstetrics and gynaecology could be possible in Europe. However, it is hoped that, if the EBCOG recommendations are implemented by all European countries, then a certain quality of training will be assured.

16

Recommendations of the European Board and College of Obstetricians and Gynaecologists for postgraduate training and assessment in obstetrics and gynaecology

J. Lansac, J. J. Amy, H. G. Bender, W. Dunlop, F. Nunes, G. Schlaeder and V. Unzeitig

This text is a collection of the proposals from the European Board of Gynaecologists and Obstetricians (EBGO) group (Chairman G. Schlaeder), adopted by the general assembly of EBGO/extended EBGO in Debrecen (Hungary) on 30 April 1993, and from the European College of Obstetricians and Gynaecologists (ECOG) group (Chairman J. Lansac), adopted by ECOG in London on 11 December 1993. It has been modified following the comments of the national societies from Belgium, Denmark, Finland, France, Germany, Greece, Ireland, Italy, the Netherlands, Norway, Portugal, Slovenia, Sweden, the UK and the European Network of trainees in Obstetrics and Gynaecology (represented by F. Nunes) and adopted by the UEMS section of Obstetrics and Gynaecology on the 5 December 1998.

MISSION

To harmonize postgraduate training in obstetrics and gynecology in Europe at the highest possible level in order to provide optimal health care in all areas encompassed by the definition of the specialty.

RECOMMENDATIONS

Recognizing that training methods differ greatly among European countries, but that fully trained specialists should be competent to practice independently in any country, the Working Party has formulated the recommendations which follow.

1 Definition of obstetrics and gynaecology

The specialty of obstetrics and gynaecology involves the supervision of, and appropriate intervention during, normal and complicated pregnancy and delivery, as well as the recognition, prevention, management and surveillance of diseases of reproductive organs and factors influencing female reproductive health. Treatment of diseases of the breast is included for the countries where gynaecologists have this responsibility.

2 Means

2.1 Entry requirements:

(1) A medical qualification recognized by the country in which training is to occur.

(2) The availability of a recognized training post.

2.2 An adequately remunerated post in a recognized training program is a basic condition. Each trainee must have a tutor appointed at the beginning of training to provide guidance and advice.

2.3 For each country, the number of training posts should reflect the national need for specialists in obstetrics and gynaecology, as well as the facilities and finance available for specialist training.

2.4 Trainees must participate in all hospital activities, such as the care of out-patients and in-patients, on-call duties (both day and night), performing deliveries and gynaecological operations and participating in educational activities, including the teaching of other health professionals. Participation in audit and clinical or basic research is recommended.

2.5 Arrangements for postgraduate training must be compatible with national employment legislation in relation to remuneration, hours of work and rights of employees in such matters as sick leave, maternity leave and compulsory military service.

2.6 Duration of training:

(1) A minimum of 5 years in an approved training program.

(2) Not more than one of these years may be spent in relevant research or in another specialty such as:

(a) Abdominal surgery;

(b) Endocrinology;

(c) Urology;

(d) Neonatal medicine;

(e) Imaging;

(f) Anesthetics;

(g) Human genetics;

(h) Pathology;

(i) Basic science, eg. physiology, anatomy.

2.7 Training should be structured throughout, with clearly defined targets to be met after specified intervals. An educational plan should be drawn up by the specialist responsible for the overall training in the department and by the tutor, in consultation with the trainee, at the beginning of each attachment and progress should be monitored regularly.

2.8 It is recommended that, if possible, part of the training should be spent in a recognized hospital in another European country.

EDUCATIONAL OBJECTIVES OF TRAINING IN OBSTETRICS AND GYNAECOLOGY

1 Aims

(1) To ensure that, at the time of appointment to a specialist post, obstetricians and gynaecologists have attained standards of knowledge and specialist skills adequate to permit them to undertake fully independent clinical practice.

(2) To encourage the acquisition, assessment and application of information and techniques in order to improve standards of practice.

(3) To encourage the updating of knowledge and skills acquired as a result of such education and training.

2 Objectives

Relating to aim (1)

(1) To define the content of the training in a syllabus reviewed regularly (Appendix 1).

(2) To define the clinical abilities which should have been acquired by the specialist in obstetrics and gynaecology.

(3) To define the personal and professional attributes which are desirable in a specialist.

(4) To organize assessment throughout the training period.

(5) To ensure that individual postgraduate training programs and assessments are supervised by a designated consultant in each training unit.

Relating to aim (2)

(1) To ensure that clinical practice is based upon sound scientific principles.

(2) To ensure that access to facilities for postgraduate training is provided for all trainees.

(3) To ensure that assessment of training reflects new developments in the specialty.

(4) To provide opportunities for recruitment into, and progress within, the specialty for junior doctors of high caliber.

Relating to aim (3)

(1) To arrange regular meetings for a critical review of new clinical and scientific developments.

(2) To publicize new developments in the specialty.

3 Assessment of training

3.1 In all European countries, approval of training and trainers should be the responsibility of a national or regional authority which has the power to withdraw recognition if necessary.

3.2 Institutions that are to be used as training centers need to be approved. In doing so, the following information should be reviewed:

(1) Annual statistics;

(2) Internal quality control and audit;

(3) Protocols of clinical management;

(4) Individual appointed tutors;

(5) Trainee's educational plan;

(6) Supervision of training;

(7) Formal and clinical teaching sessions.

Criteria for minimum clinical activity will be defined and the advice of the European Board and College of Obstetricians and Gynaecologists (EBCOG) Hospital Recognition Committee will be obtained, involving appropriate experts when necessary. EBCOG will regularly publish a list of recognized European training centers and will obtain information from the national authorities responsible for the recognition of training programs. It will then be possible to compare national criteria for accreditation and to prepare uniform advice for all European training centers.

3.3 It is necessary to assess trainees: all intending specialists should be formally evaluated at regular intervals. Progress during training should be recorded in a log book, listing procedures performed and participation in teaching programs in accordance with the recommendations of EBCOG. Use of the European log book prepared by EBCOG is recommended.

Assessment during training will be of three types:

(1) Self-assessment. Trainees should record in the log book their confidence in performing recommended procedures and their opinion of their interaction with their trainers.

(2) Formative assessment. Trainers should record in the log book at regular intervals their assessment of the trainee's competence in performing clinical tasks. The trainee's interactions with patients and colleagues should also be noted.

(3) Summative assessment. It is recommended that an intermediate assessment by the tutor should be carried out after 1 year in order to identify shortcomings needing corrective action or, if necessary, to recommend a change of speciality. Each country will be responsible for organizing its own evaluation of the training program. Emphasis should be given to evaluation during training rather than at the end.

EBCOG will obtain information from national authorities about assessment systems in use and, following consultation, will devise uniform European standards of assessment.

4 Training requirements

During training, it is essential to participate in a full range of clinical activities involving out-patient and in-patient management, as well as emergency care. The amount of experience required in individual areas of training, indicated by the numbers of procedures recommended, should not be regarded as mandatory but simply as guidelines. In addition, when training in certain ones of these techniques is not possible in an individual training center, it is acceptable to substitute some for others or to arrange a component of training in another recognized center.

Obstetrics

(1) Antenatal ultrasound examination (normal and abnormal anatomy of the fetus and high-risk pregnancies): 200 abdominal examinations.

(2) Normal labor and delivery: 100.

(3) Assisted vaginal delivery (forceps, vacuum extractor, breech): 40.

(4) Cesarean section: 40.

Diagnostic procedures

(1) Colposcopy: 50.

(2) Hysteroscopy: 25.

(3) Gynaecological ultrasound examination and early pregnany problems (principally by transvaginal ultrasound, but transabdominal experience also required): 100.

Gynecological surgery

(1) Diagnostic laparoscopy or sterilization: 40.

(2) Minor laparoscopic surgery (ectopic pregnancy, ovarian cyst): 20.

(3) Hysterectomy: 45 (abdominal 25 minimum; vaginal 15 minimum).

(4) Breast surgery, including cancer (only in those countries where this is part of gynaecological practice): 20.

Scientific communications

It is recommended that, by the end of training, each trainee has presented at least one communication or poster at a scientific meeting and published at least one scientific paper in a peer review.

ORGANIZATION OF TRAINING

1 *Postgraduate courses*

Theoretical teaching at postgraduate level should not consist entirely of a series of lectures. Meetings devoted to review and discussion of research cover only part of the theoretical syllabus. Group sessions (regional, national or European) led by a trainer, with prepared contributions from trainees, are valuable and should be organized so as to cover the required syllabus. Furthermore, all training centers should hold regular meetings for the discussion of cases and a review of morbidity and mortality, recognizing that these meetings alone cannot fulfil the needs for theoretical teaching. Trainees should be entitled to have leave for attendance at approved courses and meetings, for research work and for private study. Such arrangements should form part of the trainee's contract of employment and reasonable expenses should be met by the employer or a government agency.

2 *Duties of trainers*

Postgraduate training must encompass all of the contents of the training syllabus (Appendix 1).

Trainees should be properly supervised in their clinical practice, and all the specialists of the department should be involved in the supervision of training and teaching, which is one of the duties of all clinicians working in a training hospital.

Two fundamental elements will involve additional responsibilities and should be specified in the training program:

(1) A specialist responsible for the organization of training in the department who should:

  (a) Be designated in agreement with the head of department;

  (b) Be responsible for the educational plan and co-ordination of all postgraduate training activities of the department;

(c) Be held accountable by the accreditation authorities and be responsible for training equipment, manpower and organization;

(d) Follow and participate in the assessment of trainees and provide guidance on research projects;

(e) Provide up-to-date protocols of clinical management for the trainee at the start of the training attachment;

(f) Provide guidance on research projects;

(g) Publish annual statistics and the results of internal audits and make these available for trainees;

(h) Arrange regular staff meetings and multidisciplinary discussions in which trainees can participate actively.

(2) A tutor who should:

(a) Be responsible for the individual trainee;

(b) Supervise the trainee, co-ordinate his/her activities and progress, detect difficulties and promote corrections;

(c) Ensure that the trainee is regularly assessed (see section 3 below).

3 Rights of trainers

If trainers are to be able to meet the educational needs of trainees, their own rights should be considered. These should include:

(1) Adequate remunerated time for undertaking their training responsibilities. Trainers should expect to spend 10–20% of their time on teaching and related activities. This time should be clearly identified in their contracts of employment and defended against the demands of clinical work.

(2) Adequate remunerated time for their own continuing education.

(3) Training in educational methods by such means as attendance at national or European courses for medical trainers.

SUMMARY

(1) Trainees must have an adequately remunerated hospital post and participate in all activities of the training department.

(2) The number of training posts should reflect the country's need for specialists, as well as the country's capacity to train.

(3) The minimum duration of postgraduate training in obstetrics and gynaecology is 5 years, at least four of which must be spent in a department of obstetrics and gynecology. It is recommended that part of the training (6 months or 1 year) should take place in another European country.

(4) A specialist qualification should be granted at the end of the 5 years of training after assessment of the trainee's theoretical knowledge and practical skills.

(5) The training syllabus will be regularly updated by EBCOG (Training and Assessment Working Party).

APPENDIX 1: SYLLABUS

Definitions

(1) Knowledge: basic understanding of topics not commonly used in the clinical practice of obstetrics and gynaecology.

(2) Detailed knowledge: understanding of important aspects of topics which may be more comprehensively understood by a specialist in another discipline (e.g. geneticist, pediatrician).

(3) Comprehensive knowledge: complete understanding of topics which are important in the clinical practice of obstetrics and gynaecology.

1. BASIC SCIENCES

1.1 Anatomy

Comprehensive knowledge of the regional anatomy of the pelvis, abdomen, thorax, breast, thigh and endocrine glands, particularly in relation to surgical procedures undertaken by the obstetrician and gynaecologist.

Detailed knowledge of relevant bones, joints, muscles, blood vessels, lymphatics, nerve supply and histology.

Knowledge of cell structure.

1.2 Physiology and endocrinology

Comprehensive knowledge of human physiology and reproductive endocrinology, with particular reference to the male and female reproductive systems, pregnancy, the fetus and the neonate.

Knowledge of common physiological activities, including principles of nutrition, water, electrolytes and acid–base balance, and cell biology.

1.3 Genetics

Detailed knowledge of common inherited disorders.

Knowledge of the principles of inheritance of chromosomal and genetic disorders.

1.4 Embryology

Comprehensive knowledge of gametogenesis and fertilization, of organogenesis and the development of the embryo in all body systems, of the development of the placenta, membranes and amniotic fluid, and of structural changes in the newborn.

Detailed knowledge of common fetal malformations.

1.5 Pathology

Detailed knowledge of the cytology and histology of common conditions in relation to obstetrics and gynecology.

1.6 Statistics and epidemiology

Knowledge of how to apply statistical analysis and how to collect data. Knowledge of the setting up of clinical trials and the ability to interpret data.

1.7 Microbiology

Comprehensive knowledge of infective agents, infectious diseases and complications encountered in the practice of obstetrics and gynecology.

1.8 Biochemistry

Knowledge of the metabolism of carbohydrates, lipids, proteins and nucleic acids, the role of vitamins, minerals and enzymes, and the composition and regulation of intracellular and extracellular fluids.

1.9 Biophysics

Knowledge of the physical principles and biological effects of heat, sound and electromagnetic radiation. Understanding of the principles of laser, electrocardiography, isotopes, X-rays, ultrasound and magnetic resonance imaging.

1.10 Immunology

Knowledge of immune mechanisms and the principles of reproductive immunology.

1.11 Pharmacology

Comprehensive knowledge of the properties, pharmacodynamics, actions, interactions and hazards of pharmacological agents which are used in obstetrics and gynaecology, and particularly the principles of teratogenicity and prescribing during pregnancy and lactation.

2. CLINICAL SCIENCES

2.1 Fetal medicine

2.1.1 Normal pregnancy

Comprehensive knowledge of maternal and fetal physiology including placental function and maternofetal interactions.

Comprehensive knowledge of antenatal, intrapartum and postnatal care, including psychological guidance, obstetric analgesia and anesthesia.

2.1.2 Abnormal pregnancy

Comprehensive knowledge of all aspects of abnormality of pregnancy, labor and puerperium, together with their management.

Knowledge of fetal and neonatal diseases, neonatal resuscitation and the principles of neonatal management.

2.1.3 Maternal and perinatal mortality

Knowledge of the relevant definitions, statistics and concepts, as well as their significance.

2.1.4 Genetics

Detailed knowledge of screening for, and diagnosis and management of, fetal abnormality.

Knowledge of normal and abnormal karyotypes, the genetic causes of infertility and early abortion, as well as the ability to transmit this knowledge to patients and discuss its implications.

2.1.5 Ultrasound

Detailed knowledge of:

(a) Normal and abnormal anatomy of the fetus, placenta and amniotic fluid compartment;

(b) Fetal biometry;

(c) Estimation of gestational age;

(d) Assessment of fetal growth and behavior;

(e) Evaluation of fetal and uteroplacental blood flow;

(f) Knowledge of invasive diagnostic and therapeutic procedures.

2.1.6 Fetal monitoring

Detailed knowledge and experience of the principles and practice of all recognized methods of evaluating the conditions of the fetus before and during labor.

2.2 Gynaecology

2.2.1 General gynaecology

Comprehensive knowledge of the etiology, pathogenesis, pathophysiology, symptomatology, diagnosis and differential diagnosis of somatic and psychosomatic gynaecological diseases.

2.2.2 Gynaecological surgery

Comprehensive knowledge of all basic gynaecological procedures, including breast surgery.

Comprehensive knowledge of the complications of surgery and the principles of post-operative care.

Knowledge of more complicated procedures, for example in gynaecology and infertility.

Knowledge of the applications, techniques and complications of anesthesia, and expertise in the practice of adult resuscitation.

2.2.3 Urogynaecology

Detailed knowledge of the etiology and presentation of disorders of the female lower urinary tract.

Knowledge of the principles of investigation and of non-surgical, surgical and post-operative management.

2.2.4 Endocrinology

Comprehensive knowledge of gynaecological endocrinology and its clinical applications to the reproductive system.

2.2.5 Pediatric and adolescent gynaecology

Detailed knowledge of normal and abnormal sexual development and specific gynaecological disorders affecting young girls and adolescents.

2.2.6 Disorders of menstruation

Comprehensive knowledge of normal menstruation and the pathophysiology of menstrual disorders, their investigation and management.

2.2.7 Climacteric and postmenopausal problems

Detailed knowledge of the pathophysiology of, and psychological disturbances in, the climacteric and post-climacteric, including prevention, diagnosis and management.

2.2.8 Sexually transmitted diseases

Detailed knowledge of the epidemiology, etiology, pathology and complications of male and female sexually transmitted diseases.

2.2.9 Infertility

Comprehensive knowledge of the causes, investigations and management of female and male infertility.

Detailed knowledge of endocrine therapy and the techniques involved in assisted reproduction.

2.2.10 Family planning

Comprehensive knowledge of all methods of contraception and sterilization.

2.2.11 Induced abortion

Detailed knowledge of techniques and complications of induced abortion.

2.2.12 Psychosomatic psychosexual and stress-related disorders

Detailed knowledge of the psychopathology and management of psychosexual disorders, and the influence of stress on functional disorders such as menstrual and ovarian dysfunction, chronic pelvic pain and stress incontinence.

2.2.13 Ultrasound

Detailed knowledge of ultrasonic aspects of:

(a) Normal pelvic anatomy;

(b) Gynecological disease;

(c) Infertility;

(d) Ultrasound-guided invasive procedures.

2.3 Gynecological oncology

Comprehensive knowledge of the epidemiology, etiology, prevention, diagnostic techniques and management staging of gynecological pre-invasive and invasive carcinomas, including primary and secondary prevention and terminal care.

2.4 Ethics, law and resources

Detailed knowledge of ethical and national legal issues involved in obstetric and gynaecological practice in Europe, and the resources required to provide adequate health care in the hospital and community.

Index